A provocative manifesto that teaches you how to take control of your own health, no matter your age or circumstances—from an innovative doctor and his philosopher daughter

Dr. Alex Jadad is the creator of the Jadad scale, which has become the world's most widely used methodology to assess the quality of clinical trials, and Tamen Jadad-Garcia is a health entrepreneur and philosopher. Here they combine their expertise to uncover the medical system's unstable foundations, which condemn you to be ill. The Jadads begin this exploration with a simple question: "What is health?"

Through engaging stories and case studies, the Jadads expand the understanding of health beyond the medical industrial complex. They show how distant connections in your personal networks can influence key aspects of yourself, like your weight, anxiety, and addictions; how reliance on medications can be reduced by intentionally designing the places where you live, work, and play; and how comparisons with peers can shorten your life.

In this practical guide, the meaning of health is redefined, putting you in the driver's seat and recognizing you as the most effective evaluator. Building on data and experiences from millions of people around the world, the book reveals that a healthy life is possible even with complex chronic conditions or terminal illnesses. The Jadads explain why perceiving yourself as unhealthy might actually be fatal, and how you can monitor your true health and boost it in practically any context, no matter your cultural background or socioeconomic circumstances.

With wisdom and empathy, *Healthy No Matter What* teaches you how your natural gift of adaptability equips you to overcome any obstacle, provides actionable pointers, and shows how and when to use the medical system, so that you can thrive, regardless of the twists and turns life may take.

Alex Jadad, MD, is a physician, philosopher, educator, and innovator. A pioneer of evidence-based medicine, end-of-life care and digital health, he is the creator of the renowned Jadad scale. He leads large-scale efforts to shape the future of health and medicine, is an adviser to heads of states and multinational corporations, and is the author of twelve books and hundreds of scientific articles.

Tamen Jadad-Garcia is an entrepreneur and philosopher who builds businesses and leads strategic projects with Fortune 500 companies in healthcare, consumer goods and technology. She is the author of scientific articles and books spanning end-of-life care, love, and the future of health.

D0555576

Healthy No Matter What
Alex Jadad, MD, and Tamen Jadad-Garcia
Crown • Hardcover • 01/31/23 • $28.00/$37.99C • 9780593240823

Healthy No Matter What

Healthy
No Matter What

HOW HUMANS ARE
HARDWIRED TO ADAPT

Alex Jadad, MD & Tamen Jadad-Garcia

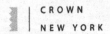

CROWN
NEW YORK

Published in the United States by Crown, an imprint of Random House, a division of Penguin Random House LLC, New York.

CROWN and the Crown colophon are registered trademarks of Penguin Random House LLC.

Hardback ISBN 978-0-593-24082-3
Ebook ISBN 978-0-593-24083-0

PRINTED IN THE UNITED STATES OF AMERICA ON ACID-FREE PAPER

crownpublishing.com

2 4 6 8 9 7 5 3 1

ScoutAutomatedPrintCode

First Edition

Illustration by Adobe Stock/arya

For the extraordinary

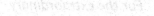

CONTENTS

Contents

For thousands of years humans tried to fly by mimicking birds. They created all sorts of contraptions, most of which centered on the ability to flap wings. All along, they overlooked the other animals and plants that were gliding and floating around them without even having wings.

This obsessive focus on one approach is exactly what each of us has been doing to achieve a long and healthy life. We are following the wrong assumptions, oblivious to the tools that we have right in front of us and persistent despite the repeated failures.

The equivalent of flapping wings is eliminating disease. Fighting illnesses through medical interventions has been the persistent method used for millennia to achieve a healthy life. This approach has made success impossible. Even by regularly exercising, eating well, getting good sleep, and meditating, we are still only scratching the surface of the possibilities to achieve this goal.

In fact, through our studies on thousands of people, we have found that 90 percent of what people need to feel healthy is actually outside of the medical system. Yet our fixation leads us to offer medical solutions to most social and emotional problems. Someone who is lonely can easily end up with a prescription for depression.

Building on data and experiences from millions of people around the world, this book presents a view of what can make a healthy and long life possible, despite the presence of disease. It is a practical guide that condenses the best scientific knowledge and insights from medicine, psychology, and sociology, going from the microscopic to the colossal.

We also underscore that you are equipped with the versatility and the tools to overcome practically any obstacle that prevents you from being healthy. At the core of all this is your natural gift of adaptation. It combines a kind of superpower and a defense mechanism that have evolved over billions of years through a practically infinite amount of trial and error. This book introduces you to this ability and offers pointers for how to put it into action.

As you go through the book, we introduce you to your lesser-known senses and ask you questions that have a highly sophisticated predictive power, including one that could predict your prospects of living or losing 20 years of life.

We also give you words to decode, describe, and deal with practically any challenge to your health in a wide range of contexts, regardless of your cultural background or socioeconomic circumstances, all based on scientific evidence.

We will show you trees that heal, pills that are labeled as fake but still work, how big cities are the best places for living past 100 years old, and why making comparisons between you and your peers can kill you.

You will learn that as much as the traditional medical system can save lives, it can also be a hotbed of lethal threats. Recognizing that it offers 10 percent of what you need to feel healthy, we provide evidence about whether, how, and when to use it, while showing you how to get the best possible results and avoid being harmed. We will peek behind many curtains and give you access to places that are traditionally reserved for insiders.

To start, we want to bring you into an exclusive room where world leaders once gathered, unaware that they were playing a part in a greater story.

Healthy No Matter What

WE GOT IT ALL WRONG

Do you know anyone who has never been to the doctor, not even as a child? How many of the people in your life have back pain, depression, high blood pressure, diabetes, or cancer? The answers to these questions illustrate a problematic situation: It is practically impossible to live a life free of illness or disease.

At first glance, it seems like there is no escape. If absence of disease is a prerequisite for being healthy, then we are set up to fail. Regardless of what we do, how much we exercise or meditate, or how well we sleep or eat, it is impossible to have a disease-free life.

If the absence of disease is the cornerstone of what qualifies as "health," then we are stuck with an impossible mission. A long and healthy life is completely out of reach for every single person on the planet. Indeed, this was the case up until 2008.

The Shake-Up

The temptation was irresistible. Hundreds of the most prominent leaders from the healthcare sector, including dozens of ministers of health, ministers of finance, ambassadors, and investors from across the planet, were assembled in a magnificent eastern European concert hall that had been turned into an elegant conference venue for a meeting held in June 2008. The agenda, which was specifically focused on the impact of health systems on people's health, had just been interrupted to celebrate the 60th anniversary of the World Health Organization (WHO).

A microphone was being used by participants to express their appreciation of and gratitude for the first institution to garner the support of all members of the United Nations. The WHO was established following World War II as a way to showcase, naïvely, how generous and caring humans could be toward one another.

As Alex approached the microphone, he could remember how disturbed he had felt a few months earlier by a question he had been asking himself persistently. It had come to him while he was recovering from an awful medical test that had finally ruled out a diagnosis of colon cancer. This was the same question he was about to ask the entire room. It was perhaps the one for which he should have had an answer, especially given that he had been either a student, physician, or professor at some of the top medical schools in the world during the past 30 years.

When he reached the microphone, he looked at the audience, paused, and asked: "What is health?"

The audience's surprise quickly turned into nervous murmuring. The moderator was clearly unsettled by the change in mood. Seizing the opportunity, and using an even more emphatic tone, Alex then asked: "What do *we* mean by health?"

The room went quiet. He waited in silence. After a few more seconds, someone stood up and said something like: "Doctor

Jadad, the definition of health appears at the beginning of the constitution of the very institution whose 60th birthday we are celebrating today!" Then the man proceeded to recite the statement that Alex had learned as a very young medical student and that had remained unchanged for six decades: "Health is a state of complete physical, mental and social well-being and not merely the absence of disease or infirmity."

Following an intentionally long pause, Alex replied with a question to everyone in the room that revealed the true intention of his inquiry: "Could you please raise your hand if you have *complete* physical, mental, *and* social well-being?"

After a few moments of self-evaluation, only one hand went up. Just one, out of thousands.

Looking at the single respondent, Alex noted that this person was the perfect exemplar; a gift for making his vital point. Alex said: "Impossible! You are wearing glasses. You have at least one eye disease."

All the moderator could say was: "Thanks for such interesting questions."

After the session, a colleague approached Alex and said: "You normally throw grenades at our meetings. This was a nuclear bomb!"

A Justified War

How could a definition of health that condemns most people to be "not healthy" have been proposed in the first place? Requiring a state of "complete physical, mental and social well-being" and not just "the absence of disease" disqualifies most people from being considered healthy. Just by having dental cavities (which occur in almost 100 percent of adults), by feeling tired or hungry, by worrying about a loved one, or by being concerned about debt or an exam, you would not be considered healthy according to this definition.

What could have possibly motivated all members of the United Nations to endorse such a view of health? An easy answer is that the WHO definition should be regarded as an aspirational gesture. It could have been inspired by the strong sense of optimism that followed the Second World War. Yet another possibility is that the definition was driven, from the beginning, by an interest in the expansion of medicine into all aspects of life.

Regardless of the initial motivation behind it, this definition of health acted as a nod of approval, an open door, to advocates of a new global war—one that was desirable and just. This war would be fought by medical professionals as its soldiers, armed with weapons created by science, produced by factories, and deployed in institutions. It would be known as "the war against disease."

The motivation of humanity to choose this path was justified, to a large extent, by a major breakthrough: the mass production of penicillin by pharmaceutical companies in the US. The use of penicillin saved at least 100,000 Allied lives during the 11 months that separated D-Day from the final German surrender. Factory-produced penicillin provided solid evidence, for the first time in history, that industrialized scientific innovation could control infections. This achievement was the first clear example of the power of combining biology and the industrial process to conquer death on a large scale. And not just any kind of death: the main cause of human death since time immemorial. At that time, worldwide life expectancy was around 45 years of age, and practically everybody knew someone who had died of "blood poisoning," caused by something as minor as a splinter or a sore throat.

The allure of penicillin, known as "the miracle drug," made it easy for the public to believe that if it was possible to defeat the most common killer, it would be even easier to eliminate all of the other threats to human well-being. As a result, most industrialized countries started to increase their expenditures on budding "healthcare systems," building hospitals and equipping them with the latest technological developments. Simultaneously, university-trained physicians became the dominant group of service providers, gaining exclusive control over the prescription of drugs and medical devices and the performance of surgical procedures.

By the end of the 20th century, this turn of events seemed more than justifiable. Medicine had successfully come up with effective ways to diagnose and repair important damage to body parts, particularly damage caused by trauma or infection. It also had succeeded in transforming many diseases that were regarded as lethal, such as diabetes and cancer, into manageable chronic conditions. Nevertheless, these gains came with consequences.

As people around the world became increasingly seduced by the promise of industrialized science to find cures for all diseases and to make "a state of complete . . . well-being" possible, medicine began to take over more and more aspects of everyday life. By the time the WHO celebrated its 60th birthday, the medical establishment had almost complete dominion over all matters related to health and illness, with its influence extending from before birth to after death. At that point, pregnancy, a natural physiological process that for centuries had been considered a normal part of family life, began to be considered a clinical condition that should be under the full control of the medical profession. As a consequence, the body of a pregnant woman became "construed as uncontrollable, uncontained, unbounded, unruly, leaky and wayward." At the other end of the spectrum of a human life, major discussions were taking place around another issue that had been regarded as normal: mourning after the death of a loved one. There were battles about whether it should be diagnosed as major depression. In the end, those who supported this medicalized view won. Subsequently, many people who were grieving became eligible to join the growing number of individuals receiving psychiatric medications.

This expansion of medicine into all aspects of life managed to reduce a large amount of suffering and even eradicate common diseases like smallpox, while simultaneously creating new ones. These accomplishments motivated and fed the growth of a "medical industrial complex," resulting in a large gain in political and economic power for those behind it. At the turn of the 21st century, this complex was consuming 10 percent of the combined GDP of the world and was feeding a vast network of pharmaceutical companies, manufacturers of medical devices, insurers, clinical institutions, and educational programs supplying products and services for a profit.

As acute diseases were being cured, chronic conditions emerged as the main targets of medical warriors. These fighters needed to acquire progressively greater levels of specialization and increasingly costly and complex weapons. This had an effect on the financial margins for investors and heightened the risk of conflict between public and private interests. The financial requirement to feed the obsessive pursuit of cures for chronic diseases led to the cannibalization or neglect of other activities. Today, the most advanced economies spend, consistently, less than 3 percent of their healthcare budgets on prevention, with most of their remaining resources going toward funding ineffective or weak treatments.

Before long, it became clear that throwing more money into the medical industrial complex was unlikely to yield new victories. The situation in the US, the country that spends the greatest amount on "disease care" services in the world, indicates that the opposite might be true. Report after report, over the years, has shown that Americans have the shortest life expectancy and the highest maternal and infant mortality rates as compared with other high-income nations.

The relentless investment of financial resources to fund the war against disease also highlighted a terrifying possibility, which has remained largely hidden from view: Medicine itself might have become the main cause of preventable deaths. In the US, perhaps the only country for which data have been collected, this seems to be the case. An understandably controversial report published in 2005 estimated that "deaths by medicine"—or the number of deaths caused by medical errors, complications from medical procedures, and adverse effects of medications—could have ranged from 780,000 to 1 million in 1999. This number is equivalent to seven full passenger jets crashing every day and exceeds by far the number of people who died of heart disease or cancer that year. Since then, medical errors and adverse effects of drugs have been ranked as the third and fourth causes of overall mortality in the country, year after year. When these two sources of mortality are added together, the number of preventable deaths they cause annually surpasses the number of American soldiers who died during the Second World War.

All these disturbing facts lead to two key questions: What needs to change? Is there a practical way to begin?

A Global Overhaul

The answer to both questions emerged just a few weeks after the 60th anniversary of the WHO: A new definition of health was needed.

It was clear that the new version could not rely on the same premises as the original one. Two foundational elements of that definition condemned us all to the ranks of the non-healthy. The first was that no one can have complete physical, mental, *and* social well-being. The second was that it is impossible to live a life absent of any disease.

Given that this new definition would have a significant impact on the life of every human being, an invitation to the entire world was issued in December 2008. The invitation was to create a new definition of health, together.

A global conversation was launched. Everyone was able to make any contribution they deemed appropriate. With the original WHO definition as the starting point, anyone could propose amendments or alternatives, challenge what was emerging, or suggest ways to enhance it.

The response was overwhelmingly positive. In the first six months, more than a thousand contributions were received from physicians, nurses, managers, researchers, policy makers, community leaders, patients, and other members of the public from more than 50 countries. As the comments were collated, it was very stimulating to see validation of the criticisms of the WHO definition, as well as references to efforts made over the ages to capture the meaning of "health" and suggestions to replace it.

This response motivated leaders to call a summit in The Hague in 2009. Alex joined inspired contributors to the global conversation, longtime critics of the WHO definition, and the host team to take this effort to the next level. During the gathering, they focused on distilling the main insights collected during the previous year. Their common objective was to transform these insights into something that would be clear, useful, and actionable by anyone, anywhere.

By the end of the meeting, there was a breakthrough. The combination of diverse views and backgrounds had paid off.

The feat of creating a new definition was accomplished through a double maneuver. First, rather than a "state," which is fragile and rigid, health should be viewed as an ability. From this perspective, it is something that you can learn, improve, assess, and monitor.

Second, instead of focusing on the unattainable goal of "the absence of disease," the new concept of health is directed at something that sets you up for success across various situations and times: adaptability. By consensus, the updated definition of health does not include the words "complete" or "disease."

Taken all together, health can now be defined as:

The ability of individuals or communities to adapt to the inevitable physical, mental, and social challenges faced throughout life.

This fundamental shift marked the beginning of a radically new way for you to make choices and to navigate the medical space, opening new possibilities for you to be healthy, no matter what.

CHAPTER 2

HOW ARE YOU FEELING?

Being healthy is like having a relationship with a loved one whom you have taken for granted, left in the background, and pushed down from the top of your priority list, often because of work and procrastination. When the bond is in jeopardy or gone, it brings a lot of suffering, with multiple regrets at the core, mostly coming from what could have been done and said but was not. Losing a relationship with someone special in your life is something you can likely relate to because of your own past experiences or those of others close to you.

When it comes to your health, how much do you think you would regret neglecting it? What if you knew that taking just 10 seconds to answer a question about how healthy you feel could point to your prospects of living or losing 20 years of life?

By the late 1990s, studies from 12 countries had already shown that just feeling that you are not healthy could actually result in your dying sooner than expected. Since then, hundreds of studies from all over the world have confirmed this. The news is not all tragic, though. Other studies have shown that you can do a lot to shape your health with what is already available to you and can even extend your "health span" (the length of life you experience as healthy). They have revealed options for improving your health that go way beyond medical interventions or trite recommendations such as those that direct you to eat well and exercise regularly.

So how do you know if you are healthy? With the old definition of health, the answer may have been to seek a medical opinion. But things have changed.

The answer now is actually surprisingly simple: You ask yourself. The process is like reviewing a stay at a hotel or a meal at a restaurant. In most cases, it is what you think that matters most. You do not have to be an expert hotelier or chef to be able to rate your experience; your assessment is independent of the professionals'.

Just pegging your health to a thumbs-up from a medical professional might be risky, since doctors are trained to find diseases. Give a doctor enough time, tools, and incentives, and they will find something amiss. This is not to say that doctors do not have an important role to play, because they do. Obviously, if you have a life-threatening condition or a serious disease, their knowledge and skills are critical for things to go well. However, in almost all other cases, being healthy is part of a bigger picture in which you hold a much more powerful position to both assess and affect your own health. The key lies in understanding that health is an ability that is mostly experienced by you. Your perspective is more valuable than you may think.

This may sound strange at first, though what is really crazy is how long we have collectively allowed others—especially healthcare professionals—to tell us how we feel. In fact, answering the following question is the easiest and most reliable way to know whether you are healthy or not:

*In general, how would you rate your health: excellent,
very good, good, fair, or poor?*

Take a second to answer this question for yourself.

Whatever option you choose is called your self-rated (or self-reported or self-assessed) level of health. This question has been used by scientists since at least the 1950s. Before that, only medical doctors had the ultimate power to deem you unhealthy, even if you felt otherwise, and there was practically no way of going against their word.

Why were doctors so dominant at that time? Physicians' power had increased substantially since the middle of the 19th century, when medicine was "professionalized." That meant medical doctors started to become the only group of people who could tell you with authority what was wrong with you, to ordain what was right for you, or to hand you a prescription. By the last quarter of the 20th century, physicians still had almost absolute power to decide what constituted a "health need" for people in general as well as for individuals. This had also positioned them as the only professionals with the authority to determine what "healthcare" must be provided to society. Consequently, members of the general public were viewed mostly as passive or inactive creatures at the bottom of a hierarchy of knowledge, with physicians at the top.

This situation started to change radically in the late 1990s, when the internet began to allow the public to bypass physicians as the gatekeepers of health knowledge and to have direct access to both the best available external evidence and their own personal clinical information. With this, fresh opportunities emerged for laypeople to free themselves from the age-old "paternalistic" or "priestly" relationship that had been imposed on them by medicine. The public now had new possibilities for their views and preferences to play a greater role in decisions about their own health.

As this practice of asking people to rate their own health expanded, thousands of studies looked at the differences in responses among age-groups, genders, ethnicities, and races, even including people enduring terminal diseases. The findings have been groundbreaking.

Rather than reading into what each response option means, two groups of responses are created with very different ramifications. If you answer "good," "very good," or "excellent" to the question, you are considered to have positive health. If you choose "poor" or "fair," you have negative health. Both groups are fascinating to dive into and try to understand better, especially because of their life-and-death implications.

Negative self-assessed health is like a fire alarm. It needs immediate attention. If you report negative health, you have twice the risk of premature death than someone who rates their health as positive. You are also more likely to become frail and lose your independence or end up in the emergency room, and you have a higher risk of practically all chronic diseases. What is even more shocking is evidence from a 2022 study showing that White adults in the US who rate their own health as poor at the age of 40 tend to live 23 years less than those who consider their health as excellent.

As different groups of people have reported their own levels of health, researchers have gradually uncovered the power of this simple question. Self-rated health can actually predict the chances of you dying of cancer with greater precision than the projections of specialists using their clinical judgment or tests such as MRIs or CT scans. Those with advanced cancer who experience their health as poor or fair have a four times higher chance of dying much earlier than those who rate their health positively.

In this way, your own lived experience is more sophisticated than any machine. It is easy to forget that humans have been fine-tuned for hundreds of thousands of years to notice changes that could be crucial to our survival, to such a point that we are hardwired to adapt. The predictive power of self-rated health is so great that, arguably, it might act as a supersensitive barometer, capable of aggregating multiple complex inputs almost instantaneously. In fact, it has been shown that whether you judge your health to be positive or negative is closely associated with more than 50 biomarkers. These indicators include fats, sugars, proteins, and markers of inflammation, among many others, which can only be detected through blood or urine tests. They show how well different organs or systems of your body are functioning. In addition to reflecting the results of clinical tests, self-reported health outperforms them in terms of estimating the risk of premature mortality.

We are all equally capable of rating our own health, but do we differ in any ways? Major disparities across groups have been found, especially along racial and ethnic lines. This is likely yet another indication of how sensitive the question is, in this case to socioeconomic and even political variables. For example, in the US, according to the Centers for Disease Control and Prevention (CDC), negative levels of self-reported health range from 10 percent among Asian Americans at the low end to 31 percent for Hispanics/Latinos at the high end. Along this spectrum, from lower to higher rates of people reporting their health to be negative, are White Americans at 13 percent, Native Pacific Islanders at 15 percent, Black Americans at 21 percent, and Native Americans at 25 percent.

Age differences are another area that deserves attention regarding the risk of negative health, which indicates difficulties in adapting. As we grow older, it is practically inevitable that we will accumulate chronic conditions, and levels of negative health increase along with the number of chronic conditions. To provide some context, the most common chronic diseases in the US among adults, according to the CDC, are heart disease, cancer, chronic lung disease, stroke, Alzheimer's disease, diabetes, and chronic kidney disease. Currently, 40 percent of American adults have been diagnosed with two or more of these diseases.

There is still hope, though. You could still feel healthy even if you have one or more chronic diseases.

Data from Canada, Germany, Sweden, and Scotland have shown, consistently, that 75 to 86 percent of people with a single disease, such as diabetes or arthritis, consider their health to be positive. The figure remains above 50 percent among people who live with three diagnosed diseases. Furthermore, a study in Australia showed that two-thirds of patients with cancer that had spread to different parts of their body assessed their health as positive, even when they knew that their disease was incurable.

Given the life-and-death implications that this self-rating question can have, we began to dig into what drives self-assessments, in order to help ensure positive health.

Why Do You Rate Your Health the Way You Do?

Just as with self-reported health, the best way to find out why people rate their health in different ways is to ask this question directly. *When you assessed your own health earlier, what went through your mind? Why did you answer the way you did?*

Researchers, including us, have asked people to think back

and try to remember what went through their minds when they assessed their own health. We looked at the views of more than 10,000 individuals from different socioeconomic backgrounds, from people in marginalized communities to corporate executives, to untangle this thought process. As expected, this exercise revealed that each person had a unique combination of reasons for their positive or negative levels of self-assessed health. Most people compared themselves to their peers, using others as reference points. What was also the same across the board was that everyone was able to quickly integrate their current and previous life experiences, personal circumstances, and expectations, taking stock of the past days, weeks, and years.

We grouped the diverse answers into themes and categories and ranked them from highest to lowest in terms of frequency to see which ones were most often mentioned. We found that the top five reasons for people to report positive levels of self-assessed health were "having a good mood" or "feeling good" (77 percent); having a strong family life and support from loved ones (51 percent); being physically fit (47 percent); enjoying a rich spiritual life with meaning and purpose (42 percent); and the absence of diseases or symptoms (41 percent).

Others who found results similar to ours decided to see whether there were differences in reasons across gender and age. They found that in general, men tend to report positive health more often than women. This is worryingly consistent. In other words, women can add this to the list of disparities they have to face. Men are also more likely than women to base their assessments on how physically fit they feel or whether they think that they can function well.

In terms of differences between age-groups, younger people who rate their health as positive are more likely to do so because they "feel fit," "feel good," and "have body/mind balance." Older people tend to focus more on the absence of physical problems or whether they are able to cope with any existing ones, as well as being able to do almost anything they regard as age-appropriate.

Clearly, when we zoom in, we can get granular and start identifying and unpacking themes and trends into increasingly specific groups. However, if we take a high-level view, a pattern emerges that is so consistent, it is almost invisible: We have never found a group with 100 percent positive self-reported health without intervention. This means that no matter who we are or where we live, negative health is a risk for us all.

Given the serious implications of reporting poor or fair health, we decided to go even further to explore what people think they need to stay healthy or to shift from negative to positive health.

What Do You Need to Maintain or Improve Your Level of Health?

We were the first researchers to try to answer this question. The opportunity came when we were approached by the leaders of a health maintenance organization (HMO) operating in Latin America. This organization was responsible for paying for the provision of healthcare services to 1.3 million people and was struggling to stay afloat financially. They presented us with the mission to figure out how to provide world-class healthcare services through a network of 35 institutions in a large city on a shoestring budget.

This seemed like an impossible task. If the HMO kept following a traditional medical model, it was clear that they would go bankrupt in less than three years. Simply tweaking how they had been doing things for the past forty years would lead to the same outcome, only a little later. We all knew that only by doing something extraordinary, together, would the organization be able to survive.

They decided to try something radically different: create a new model of healthcare. The goal was to achieve the highest possible level of self-rated health for their affiliates. And it worked. Within a year, this network managed to enable almost 89 percent of the 1.3 million people they served to experience positive levels of self-reported health by spending only about US$500 per person per year, which is almost 20 times less than what is spent in the US.

As we worked together to build this new model, every time someone reported their level of self-assessed health, we asked them to identify what they would need to maintain their level as positive or to shift it from negative to positive.

Take a second and consider the following: What would you include on your list?

Now consider your answers. How many of them would have anything to do with the healthcare system?

We answered this last question by analyzing all of the responses we got from the HMO. The findings were dramatic. In more than 90 percent of the cases, the answers had nothing to do with the medical industrial complex. Instead, the top five needs that were mentioned included the need for support to increase levels of physical activity (48 percent), change dietary habits (34 percent), deal with family issues (32 percent), improve their financial situation (24 percent), and handle some difficulty at work (23 percent). From this perspective, a marriage counselor, a financial adviser, or the head of your department at work could do more for your health than a medical doctor in most cases. If the healthcare system is needed for only up to 10 percent of cases, then a lot of the power to maintain or improve your health is in your hands.

These results also gave us an opportunity to pause and ask: Is reaching such high levels of positive health possible only because of the privilege of those who participated? To figure this out, we began another initiative to see how these findings would hold up in marginalized poor communities. This time, we dove into one of the roughest environments in Colombia.

We chose a housing megaproject on the periphery of Bogotá. Even though it is not technically a town, it has the scale and complexity of one. It contains 100,000 people from different parts of the country. Located in the south section of the capital, it has traditionally been considered a "dormitory suburb" because it offers low-cost housing options to thousands of workers in the peripheral industrial zone. The community also attracted people displaced by armed conflict and refugees from Venezuela who had been forced to leave their homeland due to economic difficulties or political reasons. With all of these factors at play, this community had very low income levels, and high rates of unemployment, crime, drug trafficking, and domestic violence.

We decided to use the same methodology as in our previous study, but this time we worked closely with community leaders rather than a corporate human resources department. Given the social, economic, and cultural conditions of the population, we adapted and expanded tools we had used previously, including the city of Santa Monica, California's Wellbeing Index, so that we could get a much richer picture of the residents' levels of health and well-being. We then trained young members of the community as data collectors. They were tasked with going door-to-door to gather information on the three core questions:

- In general, how would you rate your health: excellent, very good, good, fair, or poor?
- Why do you consider your health to be at that level?
- What do you need to maintain or improve your level of health?

Overall, 81 percent of the people reported positive levels of health, indicating how well they were adapting. Their answers about feeling and staying healthy were almost identical to those given by the other, much more affluent groups. The results were consistent, confirming that more than 90 percent of what people need to achieve or maintain positive health does not include medical interventions. However, on this occasion, lack of access to the healthcare system, even for those who did not have a medical problem, made it to the top five reasons given for negative levels of health. The ability to experience positive levels of health was, therefore, more about knowing that they could rely on the healthcare system if needed, rather than actually requiring medical interventions.

Perhaps one of the most striking findings from our research with this marginalized community was the fact that the healthiest group was young kids, especially those from 7 to 12 years of age. Ninety-six percent of them reported that they had positive health. When we asked them why, they said that they did not lack anything, especially because they spent lots of time with their parents and had love in their lives. These high levels of positive health match those in much richer countries, such as Denmark, underscoring the fact that kids do not need more money or material wealth to feel healthy. This finding also highlights the importance of interventions that could enable people to remain healthy from early childhood until the end of their lives.

Since we did that study, we have found, time and time again, that people can experience their health as "good," "very good," or "excellent" despite having incurable cancer, or when they are overburdened by multiple diseases, are under a lot of stress, are financially poor, or are socially marginalized. This can be seen as a source of hope for our ability to adapt and thrive even in the midst of the most trying situations.

CHAPTER 3

ADAPT-ABILITY

Do you ever feel that you are facing an insurmountable challenge and doubt whether you will be able to get through it? There are many inspiring examples indicating that it is possible to thrive even after having endured horrific experiences.

In the 1970s, a study was conducted on women in Israel who had been born between 1914 and 1923. This meant that they were about 16 to 25 years old in 1939, when the Second World War started. Given the timing and location of this project, the researchers decided to include a yes-or-no question about having been in a concentration camp. To their surprise, 40 percent of the women answered yes. On top of this, many of the women had also spent time in internment or displaced persons' camps, faced illegal immigration charges, and had to reestablish themselves in a country that would be involved in three subsequent wars, during which they endured an extensive period of economic austerity. Astoundingly, even after going through all that, 40 percent were deemed by physicians to be in good or excellent health and 29 percent as "functioning well." They had found a way to rebuild healthy lives and experience well-being. Many of them had raised families, worked, and established strong friendships and were actively involved in the development of their communities. Thirty-two percent of these concentration camp survivors evaluated their own overall life situation as positive. These findings are evidence of the fact that it is possible to adapt well even after enduring unspeakable suffering.

This message was echoed by a study of Vietnamese refugees in the US. They had endured a brutal war, political oppression, resettlement in overcrowded camps, separation from family members, exposure to infectious diseases, and racial discrimination, and they had seen loved ones drown or die. They experienced all of this in the approximately three decades since leaving their homeland. And yet, when probed, almost 40 percent of them reported that they perceived their own health to be positive.

The extraordinary nature of human adaptability has been revealed following large-scale natural or human-made disasters in the early 21st century as well. Katrina, one of the worst hurricanes in US history, is a case in point. By the time it hit New Orleans early in the morning of August 29, 2005, the aging levees and floodwalls had been so neglected that they collapsed in more than 50 locations. This ended up inundating 80 percent of the city, with water reaching depths of up to 15 feet. As a result, hundreds of thousands of people were trapped on the roofs of houses, in attics, in the football stadium, and in the convention center for days before they could be rescued and relocated. Despite the hardship, when researchers surveyed more than 33,000 people who were within a 21-kilometer radius from the eye of the hurricane when it made landfall, 75 percent rated their own health as positive. This was just 7 percent lower than the national level at the time.

Something even more surprising happened during the COVID-19 pandemic in 2020. As the coronavirus spread around the world, leaving in its wake increased excess deaths, high levels of stress, and mounting bankruptcies, an unexpected picture emerged. Research in France showed that the levels of self-reported health had improved twofold among people who had not been infected by April 2020, during and after the initial lockdown, in comparison with previous years. Positive health levels did not drop back down to where they had been before the pandemic; they plateaued at this new higher level, remaining stable at least until the reopening of the country later in 2020. This was the case for all occupational groups—including managers, technicians, clerks, artisans, shopkeepers, and farmers— except blue-collar workers, whose self-reported health declined during the lockdown, then returned to the usual levels within weeks after the lockdown ended. This unusual phenomenon was also described in Germany, where 32 percent of the participants in an ongoing study (which had begun in 2014) reported improvements in their levels of self-rated health during the initial months of the pandemic, with only 12 percent reporting worsening levels.

All these people around the world and at various stages in history encountered diverse threats and managed to stay healthy. This common thread shows that feeling healthy is unrelated to the type of challenges; instead, it is based on how well you can adapt in the face of adversity.

Adaptability is a subject that has been extensively studied and a term that is used within well-established academic and professional domains, especially ecology, physiology, psychology, anthropology, engineering, business administration, and management. Perhaps because of this widespread interest, the word has become part of everyday life with basically the same meaning.

In essence, adaptability is the active capacity to change in response to threats so as to become better suited to thrive under new conditions.

How Are You Already Adapt-able?

As a human, your default is to be healthy. You are constantly choosing the most efficient ways to remain so, because of your natural capacity for adaptation. You are equipped culturally, socially, psychologically, and physically to do most of your adapting without even noticing it.

To a large extent, the way in which you manage to experience positive health even under dreadful conditions reflects your ability to adapt to change itself, rather than to specific circumstances.

Some believe that humans have a prolonged childhood in order to gain the skills necessary to overcome challenges of different types and sizes. Our extended infancy gives us the skills to think flexibly and to imagine new ways to transform current difficulties into a source of strength. The reality that children face when they become adults is often very different from the one into which they were born. Childhood can, therefore, be seen as the period in which you gain the skills to deal with the inevitable "unknown unknowns" that you will find during the course of your life. This is the way in which we, as humans, prepare the next generation to lead and thrive amid changes instigated by our predecessors.

This superpower for hyper-versatility is also made possible by the strong human tendency to be connected to others, to live in groups, and to feel, think, and change together. With this, it becomes possible to co-create, use languages and other symbols, learn from one another, and benefit from imitating the ways in which others respond successfully to challenges.

Your individual and collective adaptability is also reinforced by the human capability to attribute beliefs, intents, perspectives, values, desires, emotions, and knowledge to yourself as well as to others. This has given rise to a spectacular adaptive feature: the knack for developing cultures collaboratively. As a result, these cultures can strengthen and speed up the production, accumulation, combination, and sharing of know-how in order to come up with even more diverse ways to deal with one another. Cultures can also enable us to respond in highly creative ways to known and unknown changes while transmitting those insights from generation to generation. A case in point is the creation of the tools and structures that allow us to deal with large-scale challenges seamlessly, then fade into the background with a practically invisible adaptive role. Think, for example, of elevators in tall buildings. These are key inventions that have allowed us to live in big cities. Without them, it would have been hard to attract the majority of the world's population from the countryside and to generate such a buzz of economic activity in one place. Could you imagine climbing 36 floors every time you wanted to go out for a meal at a restaurant, take a walk in a park, go to work in an office, or get some produce from a grocery store?

Essentially, we humans have evolved to be good at the "how" of dealing with adversity in its many manifestations, rather than at the "what exactly to do" in specific circumstances.

Underneath the astonishing adaptability that our human community of cultural minds gives us, we have a rich and complex biological system to deal with change. Its main advantage is that it allows us to handle an unimaginably large number of demands imperceptibly. In fact, it could be argued that if you noticed every instance in which you are physically adapting, you would be practically paralyzed. You would be overwhelmed if you focused on everything going on inside your body, even just taking one step up the stairs. In other words, the less you notice what is happening, the better.

One of the main features of this biological system for adaptation is known as homeostasis. These are the processes that maintain the stable conditions needed for you to stay alive. These include the mechanisms the body uses to keep a steady temperature as well as optimal levels of water, salt, sugar, and blood oxygen.

The notion of homeostasis stretches beyond its traditional focus on the physical body. The term has also been used to describe processes responsible for maintaining or restoring psychological, social, and ecological balance. In relation to your adaptability, homeostasis is like your internal thermostat. It operates under the radar of your awareness and keeps you automatically balanced, moment to moment.

Another key example of your built-in adaptive dexterity relates to the brain's capacity to predict what is going to happen next inside of you. This process is called allostasis. Its main goal is to optimize the supply of and demand for energy throughout the body. It is through allostasis that you are able to anticipate your body's needs and prepare to satisfy them before they arise. Allostasis is like forward thinking or proactive homeostasis. It is behind the almost immediate satisfaction produced by drinking a glass of water when you are "dying of thirst." Even though the water takes about 20 minutes to reach your bloodstream, it takes only a few seconds for you to feel less thirsty.

Crucially, allostasis is closely related to an important sense that remains largely unknown despite having been recognized since the early 1900s. It is called interoception. This is a sense that is constantly scanning the internal state of the body and sending the brain information through signals that run along nerves originating in all the organs involved in the brain's predictions. The brain, as a prediction machine, in turn uses these signals to verify the accuracy of its forecasts and to determine whether the response is right or needs to be adjusted. It has to check and double-check to ensure our survival. After all, it is encased in a dark container relying on messages coming from the outside. It is like a CEO who is locked in a room, receiving digital updates and reports from their team and in the top position to make decisions to keep the company operating at peak performance, but never stepping outside. The messages from all the divisions of the organization are equivalent to interoception in your body.

You are largely oblivious to the predictions and to most of the other mechanisms that allow the brain to budget your body's energy use. Nevertheless, you can experience the brain's responses to the many signals from the various organs. You likely call such responses being "tired" or "rested," feeling "hungry" or "full," or "needing to go to the bathroom." In this way, interoception is persistently enriching your superpower of adaptation and enhancing your capacity to anticipate, evaluate, prepare for, and respond to whatever challenges life throws at you, and your ability to assess your own health as positive, no matter what.

Your body also performs a series of mental maneuvers that contribute to the optimization of your energy use, especially when dealing with stimuli from outside your body. This is so effective that at any moment you are ignoring most of the stimuli reaching your "traditional senses"—sight, sound, smell, taste, and touch. As you are reading this book, your senses of taste, touch, and smell are practically ignored so that you can focus on your sight and on predicting what words will come next. This prevents you from becoming overwhelmed by details that could distract you from achieving your objectives as efficiently as possible. The same applies to yet another frequently overlooked sense, known as proprioception, which gives you spatial awareness.

The unnoticeability of these mechanisms—homeostasis, allostasis, interoception, exteroception, and proprioception—and your obliviousness to most of what is going on in your body, and to the challenges they are constantly managing, are themselves forms of adaptation. Erasing and ignoring parts of reality are key to your survival. You, in a way, are adapting by omission.

All these examples of how you are persistently adapting by default (of which there are many more) are outside of your focal awareness and are involuntary. You only notice when they are insufficient to deal with the challenge at hand.

What Do You Do When Your Defaults Are Not Enough?

Even when you are conscious of a challenge, you are prone to adapt. In these instances, however, almost by inertia, you tend to respond in ways that require the least amount of energy.

The response that demands the least energy is ignoring the challenge and waiting to see what happens. This is often enough to take care of it, like enduring a cramp during a jog. It is also like watching several episodes of a series or playing a video game at the end of a stressful day. In some cases, however, ignoring a challenge can lead to more harm than good. For instance, people who ignore dizziness, numbness, and slurred speech, thinking they will go away, frequently end up with serious neurological damage by unwittingly underreacting to the early signs of a stroke.

When adaptive responses lead to more harm than good, they become something else: maladaptive responses. These responses often turn the original challenge into a new problem, or even into a series of problems, with new or greater biological, psychological, or social consequences, especially in the long run. Since maladaptive responses are relatively low-energy options, the risk of catalyzing a destructive knock-on effect is always quite high. Dealing with a tendency to maladapt often requires the involvement of an experienced professional, such as a psychologist, psychiatrist, or social worker.

Another adaptive response, a level above doing nothing in terms of energy demand, is to relieve the symptoms or signs associated with a noticeable challenge. This can be something as simple as icing a sore ankle; replacing, removing, or suppressing ruminating thoughts; or eating when hungry. Along the same lines, an energy-efficient adaptive response is to focus on the challenge and try to reduce its intensity or frequency.

A more drastic, and yet highly efficient, response is to reframe the challenge. This involves mental trickery, flexibility, and creativity. Humor is a wonderful case in point. It is the most effective and most frequently used way of turning something potentially paralyzing and terrifying into something more manageable. It increases your sense of control and your bonds with others in the same context. In fact, of more than 600 paramedic respondents surveyed, 90 percent of them said that they used black humor as an adaptive strategy. The value of humor has also been shown during the treatment of cancer, as it allows patients to reassert control over the situation, gain a greater understanding of themselves and their circumstances, and get closer with the professionals involved in their care.

A higher-level response, often requiring more energy, is removing the cause or source of the challenge. This is the case when limiting activity to help mend a broken bone, leaving an overly stressful job, or ending an abusive relationship.

Adaptability, however, is not always in your hands. In many cases, it requires practically total delegation. This often happens when the challenge is acute and life-threatening. In the event of a heart attack, a stroke, major injuries from an accident, or severe pain, the only viable option is to rely on others, almost completely.

In some instances, a challenge will persist indefinitely or chronically, and the response will have to be one that can be maintained over a long period of time without becoming maladaptive. Examples of such responses include substituting a prosthesis for an amputated limb, using memory aids after a stroke, or moving in with someone to share living expenses.

Often, several adaptive responses are warranted to deal with a challenge. This is the case when a tooth infection requires painkillers to relieve suffering, dental surgery to drain an abscess, and antibiotics to kill any remaining bacteria. Conversely, multiple challenges can be addressed with one response. Parents trying to protect their kids from sunburn or skin cancer may opt for sunscreen that doubles as face and body paint. In this way, the challenges of satisfying the kids' desire to paint themselves and the parents' desire to keep their kids safe can be addressed in a single swoop, while everyone benefits.

A successful response generally mirrors the seriousness and timing of the challenge at hand. Someone with cancer, for instance, might benefit from surgery to remove a lump and cure the disease in its early stages; from chemotherapy and the relief of symptoms later if it has spread to the bones; and finally from acceptance and palliative care if it becomes incurable. Research has shown that in cases where patients must accept the inevitability of their deaths and are tasked with transferring their focus from trying to find a cure to increasing the quality of their lives, such a shift sometimes enables them to live longer.

No matter what the challenge is, if it causes you to sense your health as poor or fair (in the negative territory), the situation could be fatal. This is a signal telling you that the risk of mortality or of serious long-term consequences is high and that you must adapt quickly and effectively. In this case, the only way to achieve positive health may be with professional help (physical, mental, spiritual, or social). If, however, you feel a bit "off" but your self-reported health remains positive, you are successfully adapting, but further action is still needed.

Given that adaptability is dynamic and malleable, and that it involves feedback loops and multiple adjustments, reflection about what is happening at any moment can shed additional light on how to increase the payoff of your responses. Part of being good at adapting involves discerning the most important challenge. Initially, that may not be the most obvious one.

When you feel "off," it may be helpful to sort your challenges into categories so that you are better equipped to tackle them. Typically, the main categories of challenges are physical, psychological, and social. Physical challenges include anything related to a part of your body, ranging from something as trivial as a pimple all the way up to a malignant tumor. Psychological challenges include any disturbance in the way you think (cognitive), feel (emotional), or act (behavioral). Challenges in the social category have to do with anything negative that involves your relationships with others.

Traditionally, each challenge is slotted into one of these categories. In reality, however, a challenge can easily have aspects of all of them, with one category being more dominant than the others. A challenge is rarely purely physical, psychological, or social, and it can also vary from person to person and from time to time.

In the case of a dental infection, the main challenge for one person may be bad breath that could derail a date, for someone else the despair of losing a tooth, and for others the impact of taking time away from work while recovering from surgery or getting good pain relief.

These categories can be helpful, first and foremost, in clarifying what is going on so that you can direct your attention and efforts to getting the best support to deal with it. Second, they can improve and facilitate your communication with other people who might be in a position to support you, such as a physician, psychologist, or social services professional.

Whenever you encounter a challenge, you can parse it out and list each aspect of it under the appropriate category to the best of your ability before trying to address it, with or without help from others. Ideally, dealing with the challenge will be a reminder to you that you have enough versatility to respond to change itself and to come out stronger regardless of the situation.

Over time, no matter what you go through, you are building a history that includes all the challenges you have faced up to any given point and the ways you have faced them. That history might be innocuous or, even better, a source of joy, pride, and meaning; or it could have lingering burdensome effects. These effects can become a problem in themselves when they gain intensity, especially if they are compounded by the residual effects of overcoming other challenges. If they are left to gain strength, they can fuel the most important factor, aside from any obvious threat, that can shorten your life: the toxic stress load.

CHAPTER 4

THE TOXIC STRESS LOAD

"Give me your address, and I'll tell you how long you'll live." There is plenty of evidence supporting this shocking statement.

In 2019, a group of researchers who had compiled data about the lives of people in the 500 largest cities in the US published an alarming statistic: A baby born in the Streeterville community of Chicago in 2015 could be expected to live to 90 years old, while a baby born just eight miles away, in the Englewood neighborhood, would have a life expectancy of only 60 years. The same study showed that in 55 other cities—including New York, San Francisco, and Washington, DC—some people could expect to live 20 to 30 years longer than their neighbors. At the time, that was like comparing Monaco to the Central African Republic, the countries with the longest and shortest life expectancies in the world, respectively. But in this case, the discrepancies were found not only in the same country but in the same city. What was behind these stark differences?

The answer is something that has been hiding in plain sight for decades. We call it the toxic stress load, or TSL. This term describes the accumulation of detrimental physical and psychological changes that result from responding to challenges and exceed our capacity to adapt to these demands. It is the baggage, the scars and the tensions, collected through life, and it is the biggest threat to your adaptability. The TSL is what can ultimately kill you prematurely.

The TSL results from the combination of two main factors that influence how long and healthy your life could be. The first is toxic stress. This is the physical and psychological reaction of a person to long-term threatening situations or events, especially those that start in early childhood. The second is allostatic load, which represents the physical price paid by being exposed to prolonged toxic stress. This is the wear and tear you experience from grinding through life.

When your TSL becomes overwhelming, the response tends to be maladaptive, essentially becoming more harmful than the challenges themselves. A high TSL can trigger hormonal, immune, genetic, and metabolic changes that can be detected by laboratory tests, including those for inflammation, which can reduce the ability to fight infections or recognize cancerous cells. It can also lead to a thickening of artery walls, changes in the structure and connections of neurons in the brain, and a shortening of the tips of chromosomes. Such changes are so profound that they are equivalent to accelerated aging and might ultimately explain why people with a high TSL die earlier. Adding insult to injury, an excessive TSL is also associated with risky behaviors, such as poor eating habits, physical inactivity, tobacco smoking, excessive alcohol consumption, abuse of other drugs, and inadequate sleep patterns. Such behaviors feed the lethal cycle, contributing to a higher risk of cancer, stroke, depression, suicidal ideation, post-traumatic stress disorder, anxiety disorders, seizures, obesity, diabetes, and asthma.

Everyone Is at Risk

Nobody can go through life completely free of TSL. Its effects begin when you are inside your mother's womb and end at the time of your death. It can even be passed down to you from your ancestors, as far as three generations back, as in the case of the effects of smoking. It touches people regardless of socio-economic status, from the destitute to the ultrarich, everywhere in the world. What differs among people and communities is the intensity, duration, and frequency with which it accumulates and influences longevity and health.

Successful executives are a case in point. In terms of their resilience, work capacity, and access to most of life's comforts, top business leaders have long been notoriously vulnerable to overwhelming TSL. This risk has been exacerbated since at least the turn of the 21st century, a time of unprecedented technological development. As a result, burnout has become the norm in the corporate sector, stemming from long working hours, the intense pressure associated with making high-stakes decisions, and the reticence of boards of directors to accept any sign of vulnerability in business leaders.

Celebrities, especially top athletes and artists, are also at high risk for overwhelming TSL, as they are forced to adapt to a constant barrage of attention, public scrutiny, and lack of privacy. Part of this involves fielding harsh criticism and coping with growing expectations that they will maintain an extraordinary output. Such pressures often push celebrities to become recluses, which in turn gives rise to mistrust and isolation. In some cases, they maladapt and start relying on alcohol or other drugs, or even end their lives as a means to mitigate the excessive psychological stress produced by the "bizarre, surreal, scary, lonely, creepy, daunting, embarrassing, confusing, and invasive" world in which they live. Often, this mounting TSL becomes worse because they neglect "the truly important things"—namely, their families and oldest and closest friends.

A Stacked Deck

A lot of what happens in one's life depends to a large extent on luck. Many of the factors that influence the intensity, frequency, duration, and manageability of the TSL are already in place even before a person is aware of their own existence.

At birth, everyone is assigned labels. From that point on, these labels become practically fixed. A course is set for the intensity, frequency, and duration of the TSL that the person will experience and accumulate during their life, as well as the chances of managing it successfully.

The power of these labels is so great that each of them can lead to important differences in life expectancy and self-reported health. This is evident in the label that is assigned based on the color of a person's skin. This label began to gain importance during the European colonization of North America. Early White settlers sought to build wealth and a solid economy largely at the expense of the labor of enslaved African people and their descendants, while also eliminating Indigenous communities. This practice came into conflict with an idea that was gaining strength at the time: the universal rights of "man." The misalignment between them was resolved by manufacturing the concept of race and introducing it into law. This allowed for Black and Indigenous people to be considered as different, less than human, and innately inferior intellectually, morally, and culturally. As a result, they were formally treated as subordinate to White people.

Even though the existence of race has long been refuted scientifically, as there is no biological basis for it, people continue to be sorted and separated geographically based on the amount of pigment in their skin. This sorting has created the conditions for a self-fulfilling prophecy. Once segregation occurs, power and resources are allocated unequally, leading to disparities in income levels as well as in access to goods, services, and societal attention, which in turn feed further separation of the groups in terms of their social, economic, and environmental conditions. Such disparities are clear at the extremes of the longevity gap in Chicago. In the Englewood neighborhood, where the life expectancy was 60 years of age in 2015, 97 percent of the population was Black, and 47 percent lived below the poverty line. Meanwhile, in Streeterville, where residents were found to live 30 years longer, 78 percent of them were White or Asian (3 percent were Black), 57 percent belonged to the top 10 percent in terms of annual income, and one-third lived in homes valued at more than $500,000. The negative effects of residential segregation based on skin color were consistent with these statistics. Higher rates of premature death that could have been managed through medical interventions, greater infant mortality, and increased risks of cancer, disability, and mental disorders have been documented in Black populations consistently for decades.

The impact of residential segregation was also clear during the COVID-19 pandemic. When comparing the same two Chicago neighborhoods in 2020, researchers found that the mortality rate associated with the coronavirus in Englewood was almost 15 times higher than in Streeterville. This emerging pattern was repeated, albeit with a lesser intensity, in all regions of the country. This underscores the insight behind sayings such as "Your zip code is more important than your genetic code."

The effects of racism and segregation can easily be observed at the international level as well. Comparing countries in terms of life expectancy and the World Bank's national wealth rankings reveals that the bottom 88 nations on the World Bank's list, classified in the low-income category, have majority Black populations, and half are in Africa. When the list is viewed from the top down, the first 30 countries, which all fall in the middle- and high-income categories, have the longest life expectancy at birth and have populations that are overwhelmingly White or Asian.

The distinctions between groups perceived as racially different is also noticeable in terms of their levels of self-reported health. A national study in the US showed that after adjusting for age, sex, income level, health insurance, and health-related behaviors (e.g., drinking and smoking), African Americans were twice as likely as their White counterparts to report negative health.

How much of this difference is a result of disparities in living conditions? The answer seems to be all of it. When Black and White Americans were asked to rate their own health in integrated communities where they had the same income levels, the difference disappeared.

Along similar lines as race, though a separate issue, is ethnicity, another label that is assigned to people at birth. Like race, ethnicity is a manufactured concept. In fact, it has even deeper historical roots than race, as the word seems to have originated in ancient Greece, where it was used to identify members of "foreign" or "barbarous" groups of people.

What makes ethnicity even more effective than race in marginalizing people is the fact that members of ethnic groups in general agree that they are different, seeing themselves as sharing traditions, ancestry, language, history, religion, and culture that are distinct from those of other collectives. For example, in 1970 the US Census included "Origin or Descent: Mexican; Puerto Rican; Cuban; Central or South American; Other Spanish" as a category representing one ethnic group. As this consolidated group became the largest "visible" minority in the US, replacing the "Black/African-American" racial group in the census, the impact of a high TSL on its members became evident. The data on this group started to echo research on racial differences, revealing that members of the "Hispanic or Latino" ethnic group experience higher risks of diabetes, obesity, and a late diagnosis of cancer. They are also victims of hate-driven or bias-related violent attacks by non-Hispanic Blacks more often and have higher levels of negative self-reported health.

There is, however, a silver lining. Sometimes we are surprised when factors that are normally considered disadvantages are shown to be health protective. This is the case with the "Hispanic paradox." Research shows that Hispanic/Latino males and females in the US consistently die less frequently from heart attacks or strokes than non-Hispanic Whites, even though they have higher rates of obesity and diabetes and lower overall socioeconomic status. One possible explanation for this tantalizing statistic focuses on the high levels of social support and optimism they have. This makes them more adaptable to sources of socioeconomic or psychosocial stress.

A more interesting alternative explanation points to the role the Spanish language might play in enhancing the capacity of Hispanics/Latinos to adapt to the challenges they face. For one thing, Spanish has more words to describe positive emotions than English. Some people believe that the language also allows speakers to minimize the effects of stressful situations by using word variations that move events to "another reality" so that they can gain distance from the threats and find creative ways to avoid harm or modulate the emotional impact. For example, in English, if someone broke a glass, they would say, "I broke the glass." In Spanish, they would say, "The glass broke," protecting themselves from guilt by distancing them from the negative incident. Lastly, it has been suggested that the Spanish language contributes to a culture that yields strong social connections and promotes a happy attitude toward life in general.

Marked Cards

There is yet another manufactured factor that often compounds the power of inventions such as race and ethnicity: immigration status. This label is tied to the little-known fact that global passports to cross national borders were only invented after the First World War. Although the idea was championed by the League of Nations (the precursor of the United Nations), it was the US that executed and enforced it most aggressively. Before that time, foreigners could enter the country following a brief disease check and a few questions. After World War I, however, Congress passed a law limiting the inflow of immigrants, especially those coming from countries regarded as a threat to the future of American society. Their entry was restricted either because it was thought that they would bring diseases into the country or had a propensity to poverty, or because of their alien beliefs. From that time on, strict quotas on so-called new immigrants became the norm. These people were ranked based on the "desirability" of their national origins.

How could immigrants' origins be identified easily? By a passport, of course. This label emphasizing country of origin has long-term implications for health and adaptability. At the time people move to the US or any other wealthy host country, health disparities often do not exist. In fact, recent immigrants as a group are either as healthy as or healthier than the host population. This phenomenon is known as "the healthy immigrant effect." Over time, a change occurs, and this position of strength vanishes. This advantage is lost because of an increase in disease prevalence and premature death that matches that of the native population. In the end, discrimination and immigrants' efforts to blend in with the local culture result in a higher TSL. These consequences are associated with an increase in risky behaviors and chronic illnesses in immigrant groups. The trend is seen consistently across people from different places of origin and receiving countries, making it a global phenomenon.

Another label, albeit usually unspoken, that can have a deep influence on people's health and longevity, and which tends to persist across places and even generations, is social position. This was illustrated by a long-term study of thousands of civil servants in London that began in the late 1960s. The project, which benefited from the British obsession with class structure and the collection of data from all walks of life, produced a groundbreaking finding: People second from the top of the hierarchy had higher mortality rates from heart disease and most other major causes of premature death than those above them. Those third from the top had higher rates still. In a nutshell, the higher a person's social position, the lower their risk of developing diseases and the longer their life span.

This phenomenon, which has been labeled "the status syndrome," has been documented all over the world and cannot be explained by the usual factors, including poverty, lack of access to healthcare services, unhealthy behaviors, or traditional risk factors such as high cholesterol levels or high blood pressure. It even seems to be independent of the actual position that the person occupies in the social hierarchy. Instead, it stems from the meaning the person gives to their position, how they perceive themselves relative to others, and how much they can control events in their life and participate in society. In other words, beyond the point at which basic needs are met, it is not what a person has that matters. It is how they feel it compares with what others have, and what they can do with it.

Thus, one person's health may be made worse by another person's wealth or status. In this context, wealth and status can come from sources other than money, including fame and recognition. A study of Oscar-winning actors showed that recipients live 4 years longer than their peers. This difference is bigger than the gain in life expectancy (3.6 years) that Americans would get if heart disease were eliminated. The advantage observed among Oscar winners could not be explained by their having more money, as one of the control groups included financially successful Oscar nominees. Instead, it boiled down to appreciable status. The same effect was not found when Oscar-winning screenwriters, who are hardly recognized socially, were compared with peers who had not received an Academy Award.

Something similar is found at earlier stages in life. The impact of social status and rankings when a baby is born has been documented in relation to physical, intellectual, emotional, and social development. The message from the data is clear: The higher the social position of a family, the greater the likelihood that the children will flourish, and the better the indicators of their development will be on all measures throughout their lives.

There is yet another label with even greater power to influence how long and healthy a baby's life will be: the sex assigned at birth. Since the 1930s, when all other factors are kept equal, in every country on earth females have a longer life expectancy than males and a lower mortality rate from diseases as they grow older. The source of this longevity gap in favor of females, which has been the subject of intense debate among scientists for decades, seems to be a combination of biological, social, and behavioral factors. From the biological perspective, males appear to be naturally set from the time of birth to die earlier than females. In fact, the male fetus is more vulnerable to maternal stress and pregnancy complications, experiencing a higher rate of preterm deliveries due to a high TSL, as well as a higher rate of mortality resulting from infections and congenital disorders. Later in life, males tend to die more often and earlier from chronic illnesses.

Some of the explanations for this pattern point to genetics. One of the hypotheses focuses on the XX (female) and XY (male) chromosomes. The idea is that females are less vulnerable than males to infections or disorders while in the womb because damage to one of the X chromosomes could be easily compensated for by healthy genes on the other, which is impossible for males, who only have one X chromosome. Other studies suggest that sex hormones could also contribute to the female longevity advantage, as estrogens have protective effects against cardiovascular disease, while males have higher levels of androgen, which is associated with a greater risk of the development of such disease. This hormonal difference might also give females a greater capacity to mount stronger immune responses against infections, as compared with males.

These natural advantages for females, which have also been seen in other mammals, can be counterbalanced or boosted by important contextual and behavioral factors. An increased TSL among females generated by systematic discrimination, oppression, and segregation, combined with a reduction in risky behaviors and an increase in family involvement by males, can narrow the longevity gap between them. This started to happen toward the end of the 20th century, when the differences between the sexes began shrinking in the most affluent regions of the world.

Even though females tend to live longer, data show that they are affected by more acute and chronic conditions, as well as by more short- and long-term disabilities, than males, and that they use more healthcare services and prescription and nonprescription drugs than males, even after issues related to reproductive risks are excluded. This conundrum was resolved by studies revealing that females face greater rates of health-related problems not in spite of living longer, but *because* they live longer. In other words, they have much more time than males to develop diseases and disabilities and to seek more medical services.

The Hand Is More Than the Sum of the Cards

In addition to the labels assigned at birth, other factors can influence the TSL throughout life. These include sexual orientation, income level, educational achievements, marital status, religious affiliation, levels of physical and cognitive ability, and appearance (mainly "looks," weight, and height). In most cases, because these factors are dynamic, changing them can counteract the effects that sheer luck has on longevity and health. In other cases, they compound one another, reducing the chances that a person will enjoy positive health.

Indeed, in the 19th century, activists called attention to something that had remained overlooked: A person has multiple identities and labels that interact constantly and simultaneously, increasing or decreasing the power of privilege or disadvantage. An ethnic minority female, for example, is impacted not only by patriarchy, as a White female is, but also by the combined power of discrimination and marginalization conferred by the combination of her sex, race, and social position. This "simultaneity" of labels, which was stressed by Black American lesbian feminists in the 1970s, morphed into the term "intersectionality" in the late 1980s. It became a core framework for examining how different aspects of a person combine to create different forms of disadvantage and privilege. This led to the recognition that young uneducated females might have a higher risk of premature mortality from heart attacks than males, and that Black females who hold a college degree report worse health than White males, White females, and Black males with a high school diploma.

An intersectionality lens has also led to the discovery that premature mortality can occur all along the privilege spectrum. Death by suicide among physicians is a disturbing case in point. These professionals are at the intersection of many sources of privilege, such as high income, high education level, and high social position. Even though they benefit from lower rates of premature death from all other causes, suicide rates among them are higher than in the general population. This is a trend seen in many parts of the world. In the US alone, it is estimated that one physician dies by suicide every day. A large-scale study in Denmark showed that physicians there have a higher risk of suicide than members of any of the other 55 occupations considered. An intersectional approach makes important differences between sexes visible. Male physicians are 40 percent more likely to die by suicide, while female physicians have double the risk of ending their own lives than their non-physician female counterparts in the general population.

How many labels applied to you could be contributing to a high TSL? Which are the most problematic? Is there anything you can do about them?

It is possible that some labels you identified as a hindrance might have the opposite effect. An intersectional perspective has revealed a few encouraging paradoxes. Children of recent immigrants, for instance, are expected to be particularly vulnerable to emotional or behavioral disorders because of the stress caused by the poverty, discrimination, and social isolation typically faced by their families during resettlement. However, they fare better than children with native-born parents, regardless of whether their families are White or have a similar racial or ethnic background. Another conundrum is "the obesity paradox" among elderly people who are overweight or obese. They have a lower risk of all-cause premature mortality—particularly from stroke, cancer, heart attack, diabetes, and infection—than those with normal weight.

These paradoxes suggest that even if the deck is stacked against them, there are always ways in which any group, no matter how disadvantaged, can escape the consequences of an overwhelming TSL and avoid unhealthy behaviors, chronic diseases, and premature death. In fact, between 63 and 93 percent of people who belong to three or more marginalized groups report positive levels of self-reported health.

Winning with the Cards You Are Dealt

In addition to the many insights that emerge from studying why life expectancy can be shorter among some groups, there are many to be discovered at the other end of the spectrum, by looking at those groups that live longer.

At the outset, the most privileged groups are expected to be characterized in the opposite way to the most disadvantaged. Therefore, the group that lives the longest should include native-born, highly educated, wealthy, upper-class females who belong to a dominant racial or ethnic community and carry a passport that allows them to travel to many countries without a visa, and who live in a high-income country. This expectation is validated by real-world data. In 2021, the female citizens of Monaco had a life expectancy of 93.4 years. At the time, their home country had a GDP of more than US$190,000 per capita, with the 4th lowest infant mortality rate, the 10th most powerful passport in the world, and zero homicides per year from 2007 to 2018. The per capita income in the country had been consistently so high that the nation did not track poverty rates. Because of these indicators, Monaco might serve as an aspirational benchmark for all other countries on earth.

Other groups of people with exceptional longevity that offer potentially useful clues are those living in the so-called Blue Zones. These are regions, deemed to have "the world's longest-lived cultures and most extraordinary populations," where a higher than expected number of people live much longer than average. They include Okinawa, Japan; Sardinia, Italy; Nicoya, Costa Rica; Icaria, Greece; and a group of Seventh-day Adventists in Loma Linda, California. Supposedly, they all share some key characteristics that might be generalizable to other populations around the world.

Aside from being isolated places, with communities that draw from a somewhat related genetic pool, the Blue Zones are all places that encourage physical activity in natural settings. The people who live there put family ahead of other priorities, have a clear life purpose, have low rates of smoking, drink alcohol moderately (except for the Adventists, who are urged to abstain from alcohol altogether), eat predominantly beans and other vegetarian foods in small portions early during the day, belong to faith-based communities, engage in relaxing activities to reduce stress, and surround themselves with other people who reinforce such activities.

Studies on centenarians—people who live beyond 100 years of age—provide additional insights into longevity. They were exceedingly rare in the world before the 1800s. At that time, the odds against reaching 100 years of age were estimated to be roughly 20 million to 1. By the early 1900s, in western Europe, as life expectancy reached 40 years, the odds were 80,000 to 1. Then, between the 1950s and the 1980s, on average, the number of new centenarians increased at an annual rate of about 7 percent. Assuming that the pace of increase in longevity that began in the mid-1850s will continue, it has been estimated that most people born after 2000 in France, Germany, Italy, the UK, the US, Canada, Japan, and other countries with long life expectancies will celebrate their 100th birthdays.

Another interesting insight into longevity from centenarians is that the onset of disabilities, major diseases, and frailty is delayed until very close to the time of their deaths. Rather than escaping physical decline or age-related illnesses, centenarians experience these things slowly enough that they are counterbalanced by their capacity to adapt to the daily challenges they face.

What is so different about centenarians as compared with others born in similar conditions at the same time? Although they appear to have protective genetic, immunological, and hormonal factors special to them, or to live so long because of chance or mere luck, research on centenarians has identified several nonbiological characteristics that could improve your chances of getting to an advanced age. These characteristics include a tendency to react with low anxiety to stressful situations and, similar to people in the Blue Zones, eating small portions (caloric restriction), maintaining an ideal weight, exercising regularly, avoiding smoking and excessive drinking, being engaged in social activities, and having close friends and support systems.

"Supercentenarians"—those who live beyond 110 years of age—provide a very hopeful picture as well, even though the validity of the data gathered by researchers about them has also been questioned. A team that found 1,707 supercentenarians in 36 countries reported that the vast majority of them (90 percent) were females and 40 percent lived in the US. When the characteristics of these supercentenarians were analyzed, some surprising results emerged. The longest-lived humans were found not in isolated small towns located in remote mountainous regions or valleys, as was the case with the Blue Zones, but in cities with at least 4 million inhabitants, in warm and sunny climates, where the life expectancy at birth was already in the mid-70s or higher.

In our society's pursuit of a long life, the challenge for researchers in the 21st century will be how to protect and value the way that life is experienced. The focus will need to be on the length of the health span, not just the life span. The insights provided by those who already live long lives are encouraging.

As people get older, they tend to value health beyond the physical domain. They perceive the decline in the functionality of their bodies as an expected and normal part of the aging process, rather than as a sign of deterioration, which allows them to adjust their self-assessments of health. By changing their thresholds, they are able to consider themselves as healthy, becoming more adaptable and better able to deal with the growing number of physical and psychological challenges that emerge as life progresses. Aligned with this view, 67 to 72 percent of centenarians rate their own health as positive. In addition, those who have experienced financial problems in the past report positive health more often than those who have never been troubled by financial adversity. Even obesity in this group seems to contribute positively to self-assessed health, likely as a reflection of a positive perception of the connection between increased body weight and success, especially among people who have survived famine. Interestingly, at this stage in life, gender differences in self-reported health disappear.

Ultimately, the message that these extraordinarily long-lived people convey is encouraging. The main factors that have been found to be associated with positive health among centenarians are psychological and part of their lifestyles. Those who live the longest are better able to face challenges because they have good relationships with their children, lack feelings of loneliness, have high optimism, and believe that they can control their own health.

How do you feel you are doing on this front? Which ones do you think require more care and attention?

These findings should act as a source of inspiration to guide psychological strategies and personal decisions in earlier phases of your life, which could contribute to staving off a high TSL while also ensuring that life is experienced as healthy, regardless of how long it lasts.

CHAPTER 5

YOU ARE WHAT YOU THINK

et's do a quick experiment.

Take a couple of seconds and think of the last meal you ate. Do you remember what it was? Do you remember what it smelled like?

For the next step, you may have to put this book down. Pinch your right index finger together with your right thumb and do the same on your left hand. Squeeze them tightly, close your eyes, and take deep breaths. When you do, try to remember that last meal. By doing this, you should be able to recall the smell a lot better.

Your increased ability to experience that smell may be due to losing another key sense (your sight). It may be because you were cued to breathe and had a second chance to think about it. How does pinching your fingers together, or either of those other actions, have anything to do with the recall of a smell?

Directing you to use your hands and close your eyes was really a device to give you permission to focus on something other than your reputation for having a good or bad memory, or even on the fact that you are reading this book. This exercise created the conditions for you to notice the power of an important function of your mind, which can play a major role in your adapt-ability: attention.

Just as you have physical and social mechanisms that help you adapt, as discussed in the previous chapter, you also have psychological ones. These mechanisms are like a tool kit that can help you change your reality, to either your benefit or your detriment.

Paying Attention

What is the main source of psychological stress for people in the richest country in the history of the world? A 2019 survey of adults from all regions of the US found that for 73 percent of them, the answer is captured by a single word: money. In 2020, other surveys revealed that roughly two-thirds (62 percent) of the participants felt that they could not overcome their financial difficulties, 58 percent said that their finances were controlling their lives, and 50 percent reported that this was affecting their relationship with their families. Indeed, financial concerns have trumped health, family, and work as the main source of psychological stress for Americans since 2007, when surveys asking this question began.

Americans attribute their money-related stress to two main sources: worry about having insufficient savings for retirement (51 percent) and excessive debt (30 percent). These worries reflect one of the strongest and most closely related unpleasant emotions for humans, often called anxiety.

"Anxiety" is a word that is applied to many different experiences, and it can be difficult for most of us to put into concrete

terms. Technically speaking, anxiety is a vague sense of appre-
hension associated with focusing attention on what could be
perceived as dangerous, catastrophic, or unfortunate, in the absence of a clearly defined, known, or precise threat. In short,
anxiety is the emotion you experience whenever you feel threat-
ened when paying attention to an imaginary thing or situation.

Often, the sense of impending danger can occur out of the
blue, without any obvious trigger or source. In some cases, even
drinking a cup of coffee or entering a meeting room full of colleagues can be enough to provoke an episode of anxiety. Such
episodes typically include one or more symptoms, such as ner-
vousness, tiredness, weakness, trouble concentrating, and even
panic. A symptom is something that is felt only by the person
involved and cannot be observed by others. Episodes of anxiety
also include physical signs such as rapid breathing, restlessness,
accelerated heart rate, trembling, shaking, and increased sweating.

The money worries experienced by Americans are definitely
a source of anxiety, especially among those younger than 40
years of age, as 52 percent of them are more afraid of retirement
than death. Obviously, they are not exposed to an immediate
threat, as they have at least two decades to create a nest egg before reaching the end of their working life. Their attention is focused on a catastrophic future rather than the possibilities to
gain financial security during the next 20 years of employment.

These worries about money underscore the main difference
between anxiety and fear. Although fear is also an unpleasant
emotion, it is associated with a known, specific, or understood
threat. You would experience fear, for instance, if you were walking home and someone pointed a gun at you and asked for your
wallet. In such a situation, you would be expected to react by
following a predictable sequence. The first response is known as
"freezing," a state of hypervigilance that allows you to stop,

watch, and listen. The second is the "flight response," the urge to run away from the threat. The third is the "fight response," which results from the need to face the threat and make an attempt to neutralize or eliminate it. Lastly, if you judged that it was impossible to run and that it was senseless to fight, you would experience the "fright response," becoming passive and surrendering to the situation. In this specific case, you would hand over your wallet. Typically, at that point, the thief would leave you alone. End of story. You would certainly experience a sudden increase in your level of psychological stress. After a while, however, you would recover and continue living your life as before, possibly remembering what happened from time to time, while making an effort to ensure that it did not occur again.

Anxiety is very different from fear, as it almost always adds to your toxic stress load. When it gets too intense, frequent, or prolonged, it can become overwhelming and even deadly. This is illustrated clearly by being overfocused on money worries. Those who face unmanageable personal unsecured debt—mostly from credit cards, mortgages, or car or student loans—have an eightfold increase in the odds of death by suicide or drug overdose, and a fourfold increase in psychotic disorders.

Nevertheless, occasional anxiety is to be expected as part of an ordinary life. It might be associated with uncertainty around retirement, struggles with debt, or events such as the first day of school, a job interview, or a presentation to a group. In many cases, however, anxiety does not go away for months, can worsen over time, and has negative effects on all aspects of daily life. When this happens, the person who experiences it is deemed to have an "anxiety disorder," something that has been estimated to occur in about 11 percent of people around the world in any given year and in 17 percent of people at some point during their lives.

The frequency of anxiety disorders varies across regions of the world, with the highest frequency in North America and the lowest in East Asia. Females are almost twice as likely to be affected as males, a pattern that persists over time and across settings with different levels of wealth. Regardless of culture, people under the age of 35 are particularly vulnerable. Anxiety disorders are also very common among people with other health problems, especially those with cancer (up to 80 percent) and drug addictions (50 percent). In half of the cases, anxiety disorders are accompanied by other mental disorders.

Given the large number of people affected by anxiety disorders, the limited number of trained therapists available, and the persistent stigmatization of mental illness around the world, it is unsurprising that only around one-quarter of those experiencing them receive some sort of care (either psychotherapy or medication). Of those, the vast majority receive medication prescribed by a general practitioner in a primary care setting, with either no benefit or only slight improvement in their condition.

Remembering that anxiety is an emotion opens up a range of possibilities to enhance adaptability.

Refocusing Emotions

A little-known fact is that emotions, contrary to what has been traditionally believed, are not hardwired into special circuits in the brain that have evolved to enable us to survive. There is no such thing as a "fear circuit" or an "anxiety circuit," which would allow us to anticipate danger and would initiate reliable physical responses (e.g., high heart rate, sweaty palms, or muscle tension). In fact, emotions are not things that happen to us. Instead, they are learned and constructed by our minds.

When you face a challenge, your brain uses messages from your traditional senses (sight, smell, hearing, touch, and taste); from your organs, through interoception (e.g., an accelerated heart rate or rapid breathing from the heart or lungs); and from your past experiences to give meaning to what it feels. This interpretation is done in the moment, informed by a lifetime of learning, and is expressed as an emotion with a label.

Anxiety, just like fear, may have deep evolutionary roots. When early humans were exposed to dangerous, potentially lethal events, it was more favorable to their survival to label unpleasant sensations as serious threats rather than to downplay them, ignore them, or even view them as the source of constructive experience. When a bush was rustling near a watering hole, some early humans might have perceived it as the effect of a pleasant, refreshing breeze, while others may have detected it as a sign of a hungry predator. In the long run, those who thought it was the latter would have had a greater chance to survive and procreate. Anxiety, in particular, has adaptive value. It prepares the body to face a peril rather than to try to escape from it. In essence, we are the descendants of the paranoid.

In modern affluent societies, the threats themselves are much less lethal. Instead, what could kill you is paying too much attention to non-life-threatening challenges, seeing them as mortal dangers. With many technological and social developments occurring quickly, and such high levels of uncertainty about these developments, negative defaults can lead to high levels of TSL and become malignant. The worst cases are those in which the worry about becoming anxious turns into a self-fulfilling prophecy, which in turn feeds a cycle that gets increasingly difficult to break. When you become anxious about being anxious, you pay a hefty price.

How can you adapt to challenges like these, which bring

about so many unpleasant emotions? Fortunately, all the intense sensations we experience when we are anxious can be associated with more than one emotion. Therefore, focusing your attention on all of the physical sensations that would normally be lumped under the label "anxiety" can help you untangle them. Once you have separated them, it is easier to recategorize them under more constructive labels. For instance, an increased heart rate could be labeled as excitement, a pounding in your chest as exhilaration.

Curiosity, as absurd as it may sound, can be a good alternative. In this way, you can view the excitement of the pursuit of new knowledge as the source of any physical change you experience in relation to the "unknown unknowns" of life.

The central idea is that you have the opportunity to reflect upon what you are experiencing, then choose an emotion with a label that does not shorten your life span. You have a lot of control over the concepts that you will ultimately use to name what you are feeling and to drive your actions.

The bottom line is that anxiety does not really exist as an objective thing. As a concept that was created by people to describe a bunch of intense sensations associated with imaginary threats, it can be unpacked and reassembled into something pleasant or at least more constructive.

Overpowering Dread

Although some people might benefit from the support available through the medical industrial complex, and some others might be able to deconstruct and repackage what they feel themselves, the vast majority of people need additional support to deal with unpleasant emotions that add to their TSL. What can be done about this? The good news is that massive demand and lack of support have instigated the development of easy-to-implement, relatively simple, inexpensive, and effective measures, which can be used almost anywhere, by anyone, and without the participation of a healthcare professional, the need for sophisticated infrastructure, or even much mental effort. These approaches also have the ability to help mitigate other everyday factors that contribute to a harmful TSL.

One of the most promising options that has emerged is known as "cognitive bias modification" (CBM). The name says it all. The aim of these interventions is to change biases (unconscious faulty ways of thinking), which are the crux of anxiety. They are what make people with anxiety notice, focus on, and interpret information in such a way that it is associated with potential threats, even if it is harmless or irrelevant. These biases ultimately affect the decisions and judgments people make.

How and why does CBM work so well? It targets two types of bias that are most closely related to anxiety disorders: attention bias and interpretation bias.

Attention bias is the tendency to give priority to, process, and overfocus on negative information about the future, while undervaluing or ignoring benign or neutral alternatives. Interpretation bias refers to the propensity that people with anxiety disorders have to consistently judge ambiguous information in everyday life (actions or comments from others, words or images that are vague and could mean different things) as threatening or catastrophic.

The way CBM works to overcome these biases is very straightforward in practice. Those being treated are presented with repeated tasks that need to be processed quickly over a few minutes, with minimal instructions, and performed using digital devices. These tasks are like drills to build new habits and override harmful old ones. They are designed to improve the ability of people to shift their attention from negative to positive information, or to develop the natural tendency to assess things as positive, while rejecting threatening thought patterns, especially in ambiguous situations. This is like making it a habit to focus on the trees, plants, sky, or anything else that is beautiful in your surroundings, seeing your reality in a positive light, rather than, for example, on the potholes or traffic on your way home from work.

What would this look like in practice? A commonly used exercise to counteract negatively biased attention is based on digital images. The task for those being treated is simply to identify the location of a smiling face among a collection of angry faces as quickly as possible, and then to repeat the task with a certain number of variations over a set period of time.

Exercises to offset negatively biased interpretations are usually conducted using ambiguous images or scenarios where choice matters. The person doing the activity is asked to practice interpreting and resolving the situation in a neutral or constructive way. An exercise based on ambiguous sentences can be as simple as presenting the person with a word conveying either a threat interpretation (e.g., "embarrassing") or a positive interpretation (e.g., "amusing"). The system then shows the person a vague statement such as "After you said something, people laughed." The person is asked to decide whether the word is relevant or irrelevant to the sentence. The system responds with "Correct!" to a positive interpretation (in this case "amusing") or "Incorrect!" to a threatening one ("embarrassing").

Surprisingly, even though there are a wide variety of forms that CBM can take and many ways in which it can be administered, it is effective. An in-depth analysis of data from thousands of people found that these kinds of exercises are consistently able to modify interpretation bias and relieve anxiety disorders. Growing evidence shows that minimal, inexpensive, and highly scalable interventions can have beneficial effects, which is encouraging. These approaches are paving the way for other options that could fill the massive gap between what is needed and what is available.

BASKing in Positivity

One of the main insights from research on CBM is that by repeating behaviors, albeit very simple ones, it is possible to change undesirable responses. What has become clear is that through this kind of repetition, it is possible to counterbalance harmful attitudes that feed negative responses to external information, without requiring direct professional involvement. This core goal is shared by other promising interventions that could curb the burden of unpleasant emotions. We call the combination of their most effective components BASK:

Behavioral tasks
Attitude changes
Skill development
Knowledge acquisition

Doing physical exercise is a good example. Aerobic routines and resistance training (squats, push-ups, bench presses) seem to be most effective in curbing the tendency to label sensations as anxiety. What appears to underlie the positive effects of exercise is how it makes the body feel and what it makes the body do. In short, moving your body mimics many of the interoceptive signals that are associated with anxiety and its responses (increased heart rate, muscle tension, shortness of breath, sweating). This creates the opportunity to train the brain to favor the interpretation of these feelings as discomforting but not catastrophic. In addition, research has revealed that exercise can trigger the release of neurotransmitters, endorphins, and hormones that have effects similar to those of many drugs used for anxiety and mood improvement. Thus, even doing something as simple as jumping jacks can be a very effective "in the moment" way to feel better.

Along these lines, yoga appears to produce positive effects through mechanisms similar to those associated with physical exercise. A diverse group of randomized controlled trials on different types of yoga—mostly based on poses and sequences (asanas and vinyasas) demonstrated by certified instructors in sessions from 10 minutes to 2 hours—have shown that yoga has positive effects in children (3 years of age and up) and adolescents, especially after nine weeks of sessions. Among adults older than 30 years of age, yoga is most impactful for those with elevated levels of anxiety and without a formal clinical diagnosis of an anxiety disorder. Yoga has also been shown effective at relieving anger, especially among elderly people.

A closely related group of interventions involves mindfulness, or psychological exercises designed to enable those who practice them to become intentionally aware of their thoughts and actions while noticing unfolding experiences, without prejudice, a moment at a time. Each moment lasts, on average, around three seconds, with a longer duration for experienced meditators. Mindfulness interventions, which are based on scientific and ancestral knowledge, can help you develop the skills to disengage from dysfunctional attitudes. They push you to pay attention to what is happening, at every moment, on purpose and without judgment. Although most of the mindfulness modalities used to tackle anxiety disorders require weeks of training with a professional, there is evidence that just a one-hour session followed by a three-minute breathing exercise practiced at home might be just as effective.

In response to the lack of resources to help people cope with anxiety and other unpleasant emotions, clinic-based treatments are also being adapted to be simpler and more widely available. They have become so easy to use that they do not require professional involvement and can be administered through virtual means. The growing demand for this kind of help, paired with data showing consistently that 76 to 90 percent of people prefer virtual treatment via a digital system over therapy provided by a person, has boosted their availability and the speed at which they are being developed.

A very popular option is internet-based cognitive behavioral therapy (iCBT), which is administered through digital devices and without professional guidance. It can produce results similar to those obtained through face-to-face CBT supervised by an experienced therapist. Even more astounding are the lasting effects of iCBT. After 9 to 12 weeks of treatment, the benefits are sustained for at least 6 months.

Relaxation techniques as varied as progressive muscle relaxation, guided imagery, deep breathing, and meditation can be as effective as CBT at relieving agoraphobia, as well as fear of spiders, fear of flying, and fear of public speaking.

There are also some impressive results from the use of virtual reality (VR) involving all of the BASK components. VR achieves significant and long-lasting beneficial effects by immersing people in realistic scenarios where they are exposed to situations that trigger their anxiety. This has been shown to be particularly effective for anxiety involving phobias (fear of spiders, heights, school, dentists), panic attacks, public speaking, or musical performances. The positive impacts are comparable to those produced by in-person treatment and can last up to 6 years.

VR could be extended to offer practically every type of intervention aimed at relieving unpleasant emotions. This is illustrated by the successful results that have been shown in relation to using mindfulness for the relief of anxiety, sadness, and anger.

The use of digital means to transform negative emotions is opening the door to myriad opportunities in the so-called metaverse. This term was coined in the early 1990s to describe a digital world that is layered over the one we inhabit physically, using augmented reality and VR, where you can experience your own sense of presence while also participating in all kinds of shared activities with an unlimited number of people at the same time.

Fabricating a Healthy Reality

Your mind has a practically unlimited capacity to create reality, regardless of whether it happens in the physical or digital world. Just as it is able to fabricate scenarios of the future that can fill you with anxiety, fear, and sadness, it can create settings in which you feel calm, confident, and joyful.

Your mind can also build the conditions to change who you think you are. This is possible thanks to a sense known as "self-perception." It allows you to assess your life and determine who you are by witnessing your own actions. Think of it as an everyday out-of-body experience.

For years, it was believed that people's actions are a reflection of their personality and attitudes. For instance, a person with "a generous nature" will manifest this through their engagement in volunteer work or by donating money to charity. Extensive documentation and analysis have shown that this also works in re-verse. If a person does volunteer work or donates money, they will conclude that they are themselves generous.

Taken together, all of this, to a large extent, boils down to a very simple sentence: You are what you think you are, based on what you do. With this having been confirmed by hundreds of experiments, there is room to "make" your "self" through behaviors. Ultimately, the way you behave influences how you build your life, who you believe you are, and the world you inhabit.

In 1979, a group of 70-year-old American men arrived at the doorstep of a portal in time. From the outside, it looked like a converted monastery, but inside it was set up to simulate a regular day in 1959. Before the men—a couple stooped over and others walking with canes—entered the building, they were asked to reminisce about that year. Tasked with making a serious attempt to be the person they were 20 years before, they were treated as such from the moment they crossed the threshold. During the five days of their stay in this alternate reality, they re-created and relived their youthful pasts, read news and watched television programs from 1959, and spoke of events of that time in the present tense. To bolster the effect, there were no mirrors, no modern-day clothing, and no recent photographs. Instead, if they wanted, they could see portraits of their much younger selves.

Before entering this environment, the men were evaluated on measures such as dexterity, grip strength, flexibility, hearing, vision, memory, and cognition. The researchers running the study had also evaluated a control group that had stayed at the house earlier but did not imagine themselves younger and were not cued in terms of their behavior. All they were tasked with was reminiscing about that time in their lives.

At the end of the five days, the test group was assessed again.

On several measures, they outperformed the control group. They were found to be suppler, showed greater manual dexterity, and sat taller. Even a group of independent judges said they looked younger. The most astounding result was that their sight improved. Instructed to think that they were younger, these men behaved younger and, in several ways, became younger.

Even though the potential impact of this "fake it until you make it" approach is huge, it has limits, determined by your genetic inheritance; by the labels you were given at birth; and by the specific historical, social, geographic, and cultural conditions in which your life unfolds. Given these constraints, at least in theory you, or anyone else, can create a healthy persona by behaving like a "healthy person." Even if you do not feel like one, acting as if you are thriving in response to the challenges you face can create a world of difference.

So it is clear that it is possible, within reasonable boundaries, to create your own reality and your own self, on a daily basis, with meaningful benefits. It could be argued that it is also necessary to do so in order to adapt to the challenges you face.

Besides creating a favorable reality with the aid of digital tools or through changes in your behavior, there is yet another method, known as "realistic optimism," that can stand alone or be incorporated into the other modalities. This means having the disposition to anticipate positive outcomes while also judging whether the you would like to occur are likely to happen given your circumstances.

Realistic optimism can have many beneficial adaptive benefits, especially when someone is trying to avoid entering the medical system, as illustrated by a group of researchers who have been studying more than 22,000 Americans every 2 years since 1992. When they looked at the relationship between stroke and optimism, they were astounded. To get their baseline, they chose a starting group that did not have a history of stroke and asked them to answer three questions on optimism using a 6-point scale. They found that each unit increase in optimism—within a range of 3 to 18 units—was associated with a 9 percent reduction in risk of stroke within 2 years, even after controlling for other potential risk factors. In other words, optimism alone could protect you from stroke. Similarly, patients with lung cancer who had been classified as having an optimistic attitude up to 18 years before their diagnosis survived an average of 6 months longer compared with patients with a pessimistic attitude.

Many more studies underscore the health impacts of optimism. Altogether, they show that optimists tend to engage more often than pessimists in healthy behaviors such as exercising and eating nutritious diets, and they are less likely to smoke or drink alcohol in excess. Optimism is also associated with proactive strategies that can improve adaptability, including problem-focused coping and seeking social support, which are linked with a reduced risk of chronic disease, as well as with better psychological and physical function later in life.

Another approach to self-creation builds on the hypothesis that we are what we imagine we are. According to this perspective, you can create a healthy reality for your life by changing the stories you tell yourself about yourself. To do this successfully, it is necessary to activate the capacity for mental trickery. In a way, this is similar to the creativity that enables authors of fiction to write compelling stories, your ability as a reader to immerse yourself in imagined scenarios, and an actor's talent to embody a character. When you apply this to your own ability to adapt, you play the starring role in the story of your life and continue to write that story. In this way, you can direct the narrative toward new ways of understanding and calibrating your actions to replace self-defeating maladaptive patterns with healthy alternatives.

In light of this information, what new reality could you create for yourself to overcome your most pressing challenges?

It is also possible to fabricate a healthy reality for yourself by changing expectations. A shift in your beliefs about how future events will unfold can influence your ability to adapt to upcoming challenges and also have a profound effect on whether that reality actually transpires.

There is hardly a better source of evidence to demonstrate this than what has been revealed by experiments using placebos. These are interventions that produce effects because their recipients expect them to work. Their power, which remains unexplained, is immense. Placebos are able to reproduce and match the outcomes associated with any "active" intervention with which they are compared. In other words, a pill, cream, or injection without a drug in it can be just as effective as the real treatment.

The placebo effect is stronger when neither the person who gives a placebo nor the person who receives it is aware of it. Although this is more frequently acknowledged to happen in situations where the outcome is almost exclusively subjective, such as pain or anxiety, placebos have produced shocking results in studies that are normally considered to be highly objective, such as those evaluating the effects of surgery. In 2014, scientists analyzed 53 different trials that compared groups of patients who had undergone either "real" or "sham" surgeries. They found that in a high proportion of sham surgeries, there was improvement after undergoing the procedure. In many cases, the effect of the placebo was the same as that of the real operation.

The power of placebos is so great that in some cases, even if people are told that they are receiving one, they still experience significant benefits. For example, a group of patients with irritable bowel syndrome (IBS) received open-label placebo pills presented as "placebo pills made of an inert substance, like sugar pills, that have been shown in clinical studies to produce significant improvement in IBS symptoms through mind-body self-healing processes." Even though all the participants in the study received the same quality of interaction with healthcare providers, the patients who were aware that they were taking a placebo had better results than those who received no treatment.

Given the diverse yet consistent effects of placebos, they are considered to be a surrogate marker for everything that surrounds a treatment itself—the reality in which the placebo is being used. The impact of placebos represents the power of rituals, spaces, and interactions to enhance or protect health.

Above all, the placebo effect and the effect of our expectations about how things will turn out underscore the myriad factors hidden in plain sight that shape human health but are not intuitively or purposefully designed for medical or healing purposes. A large group of them are physical and are embedded in the very spaces that surround us. In all cases, they are human creations, which can be deconstructed, reconfigured, replaced, reimagined, and re-created to boost your adaptability and, ultimately, your longevity.

CHAPTER 6

SPACES MATTER

Imagine you are in a forest. Slowly walking; nowhere to be in the next while. Without a destination or ultimate direction. You are free to wander. You are taking quality time for yourself.

You look up and notice that you are under a canopy of bright green leaves. Some are slightly faded; others are deep green. Their edges are all different. They can be jagged, smooth, broken, or bitten. Speckles of sunlight shine through a few of them, making them seem almost translucent. There are rays of light streaking across the path ahead. You trace them back to their origin and can see the blue sky peering through. Do you see a cloud drift by or birds gliding overhead?

Your eyes work their way through the branches and leaves, down the trunks of the trees, noticing the textures. Following the canyons in the bark downward, your gaze hops from one peak to another and flows along the troughs.

You hear a little rustling in the leaves above. Some birds are scanning the panorama, taking a rest from soaring.

You notice yourself breathing. Taking a deep breath in through your nose to smell the subtle combination of classical elements: a bit of life-nurturing earth, water, and air, all warmed by the sun. Letting the breath out through your mouth.

The sound of your steps on the ground begins to quiet. You find your feet barely moving. You feel the earth pushing you up by your soles. You are standing there taking in all the life that surrounds you.

You notice a small stream close by. You can hear the water running over the rocks and through the fallen branches. You can see it now. You notice the white of the water in its movement over the rocks, the mirage-like green and brown hues from the plants, the deep black from the miniature underwater caves, the gray from the pebbles and stones. How many colors could there be in this water? There goes a water strider, doing the breast-stroke in its element.

You come a bit closer to the edge and hold on to a tree for stability. It is slightly moist and yet solid. You can trust it. The rush of the water is at the forefront of all the other sounds you can hear.

You are back now, with a book in front of you, in a space meant for reading at this moment.

Healing Nature

What you just experienced was a simulation, in your mind, of a Japanese practice called *shinrin-yoku* (forest bathing), an activity that is about being present: turning off or putting away your electronic devices; moving slowly; allowing yourself the time and space to begin seeing, smelling, feeling, and hearing everything around you more deeply, at various scales; noticing the details and the discrete features of the tiniest things that activate your senses, as well as the massive elements that inspire awe. Your breath can become consciously fuller.

What research on forest bathing tells us, consistently, is that this practice offers benefits that align with the reduction of our toxic stress load. Although the ideal amount of time appears to be 2 hours per month with expert guidance, it has been found that just standing in a forest setting for 15 minutes is enough to produce a significant reduction in anxiety when compared with the same amount of time spent watching a cityscape.

Study after study in adults has concluded that forest bathing seems particularly effective in reducing stress associated with school, work, and the use of technological devices. In most cases, it can improve mood levels and sleep quality, even in people with mild depression, addiction, or post-traumatic stress disorder. Although more limited in size, the evidence in children and adolescents indicates benefits, especially in cases of mood and attention disorders, bronchial asthma, and dermatitis. Forest bathing seems to have positive effects on biological markers of stress (cortisol levels, heart rate variability, changes in blood pressure), on the immune system, and even on brain function.

Forests are just one of many natural spaces that can influence TSL and positive health levels. Researchers have included them in a category called Green Spaces, together with any other places that allow for immersion in areas of grass, trees, or other vegetation—literally, green spaces. Parks and natural preserves are great examples. People who live close to, use, and visit Green Spaces feel healthier: People who spend at least 2 hours a week in a Green Space are 10 percent more likely to report positive health than those who do not. Astoundingly, Green Spaces have also been associated with a 31 percent reduction in the odds of premature death from all causes.

Do these outcomes apply to all Green Spaces? No. Trees

seem to be the feature that provides the strongest health boost, especially among younger people. A long-term project that followed 3,568 students between the ages of 9 and 15 from 31 different schools in London found that kids who spent more time in woodlands—rather than grasslands—had higher scores for cognitive development and a lower risk of emotional and behavioral problems.

The potential large-scale health benefits of Green Spaces are such that several countries—including Scotland, England, and New Zealand—began encouraging healthcare professionals to issue Green Prescriptions (GRxs), especially to people living with, or at risk of developing, chronic diseases.

Another group of natural settings is known as Blue Spaces. Yes, these are spaces related to water, including lakes, oceans, rivers, and other outdoor water bodies or courses, either natural or man-made, whether they are used for recreational or aesthetic purposes. But in order to be beneficial, they must be accessible to people, and you must be close enough to be able to sense the water.

Although Blue Spaces receive less attention than Green Spaces, there is consistent evidence of positive associations between them and mental and physical outcomes. People living near or having views of the coast rate their health more positively and are generally healthier both mentally and physically than those living inland. They experience fewer symptoms of mental distress and are more satisfied with their lives.

Why do natural spaces have such an influence on human health? There are likely at least two mechanisms responsible. One is derived from what is known as the "biophilia hypothesis." This perspective suggests that because humanity has relied on nature for survival and reproduction during 99.9 percent of its history, people have developed an innate tendency to prefer being close to nature. We respond positively to places that evoke those environments that used to provide shelter and food. Therefore, people tend to choose natural spaces as their top choices to feel relaxed, forget their worries, and reflect on personal matters.

Another related perspective is called the "stress recovery theory." This idea is based on the belief that nature can play an important role in reducing the TSL. The theory proposes that by visiting natural environments, people can get away from the sources of stress they typically face in built-up urban settings, and their adaptive energy can be restored. Such restoration is facilitated by the way in which natural environments evoke the survival benefits humanity has received from nature for eons. In other words, just as natural settings contributed to the well-being and survival of early humans, today they can generate feelings of pleasure and calm in us, help block out negative emotions, and provide a distraction from sources of everyday stress.

Since most people in high-income countries spend 80 to 90 percent of their time indoors, scientists have examined other possibilities for people to reduce their TSL and to experience positive health in enclosed spaces.

Creating Spaces

Green Spaces and Blue Spaces are just the beginning of a range of spaces that have been ascribed colors of the rainbow.

Another area where you can restore your depleted adaptability builds on the idea of the Orange Economy, also known as the Creative Economy. This is the group of sectors whose main purpose is the production and marketing of cultural, artistic, or patrimonial content. The places where these sectors operate can be called Orange Spaces. They are dedicated to the performing, visual, and gastronomic arts; to literature, design, gaming, and sports; and even to online, digital, and electronic creative activities.

There is increasing evidence to suggest that cultural participation enhances human health and well-being through a rich menu of options that range from witnessing and experiencing, all the way to engaging in the creative activities themselves. Just visiting a museum can curb the TSL by reducing social isolation and anxiety, increasing positive emotions (e.g., optimism, hope, and enjoyment), boosting self-esteem, and strengthening a positive sense of identity.

Women visiting art exhibitions or going to the theater, movies, or concerts at least once a month report positive health more frequently than those who are less frequently engaged in these activities. Interestingly, without a clear explanation, this effect has not been found among men.

To continue with our color guide, another group of built environments are what we call Violet Spaces, which include offices, residences, retail spaces, and educational institutions. In these spaces, the health potential ranges widely from fulfilling basic human needs such as shelter to encouraging higher-order self-actualization within a workplace or school. These spaces have features that allow you to control many variables, like temperature, noise, lighting, and level of crowding, all of which can have a strong impact on self-reported health and the TSL.

Research on office interior design illustrates how all these elements come together. Some data reveal the harmful side of open-plan offices. Shared workspaces with six or more occupants are associated with higher use of sick leave and deterioration of relations among co-workers, with occupants reporting more stress and physical health complaints. The same is true for work settings that are exposed to high levels of noise.

Some scholars and designers believe that the effect of the built environment on health is rooted in the capacity of these spaces to actually change behavior. How? Architecture seems to have a bodily connection to people, in such a way that buildings orchestrate the possible movements within them and the actions that can be performed there. These spaces establish a form of unwritten code of conduct, inducing appropriate behaviors and limiting others.

Such thinking has led to a construction boom within the education sector that seeks to transform the ways in which highly adaptable schools are designed to boost the capacity of 21st-century learners to communicate, collaborate, think critically, and be creative. Somehow, the design briefs for learning spaces historically have lacked explicit elements aimed at increasing the ability of children and adolescents to adapt to the inevitable challenges they will face throughout their lives.

So how do these Violet Spaces affect our health? Physical constructions can influence health by increasing the degree of personal control they afford people. Buildings have been shown to have the ability to make those inside them feel either empowered or, in some cases of poor design, helpless.

Studies of the latter cases, such as high-rises with multiple dwellings, have found that such units are psychologically harmful to mothers with young children and possibly to young children themselves, especially when they are members of low-income families. The two main reasons for this are that the spaces create a default of social isolation for mothers and restrict play opportunities for children, who tend to be kept inside their apartments for long periods of time. These built-in limitations often lead to heightened intrafamilial conflict and reduced opportunities for parents and children to get to know their neighbors, further fueling their TSL.

Later in life, as longevity increases, Violet Spaces can play a part in promoting or hindering healthy aging. Sadly, the pace of innovation in this area, for this demographic, is very slow. The number of endeavors that focus on the effects of the design of senior living residences with an emphasis on stress or health is not only very small but also uninspired. "Innovation" in this space goes no further than reporting how rates of positive health are higher when residences offer their dwellers a gym, a swimming pool, and a music room large enough for dancing.

So how can we break through the apparent lifelessness of Violet Spaces, which have fallen short in design features that can boost people's capacity to reduce their TSL or maximize levels of positive health?

This is where White Spaces come in. This term is reserved for those places that do not yet exist but that could exist in the future. Did you not see the green of the leaves while forest bathing at the start of this chapter? You were in a White Space, where it is possible to reimagine where we can spend our lives.

White Spaces are places of imagination and simulation, where openness, flexibility, autonomy, playfulness, humor, willingness to take risks, and perseverance are the norm. They are designed for what-if questions that are highly experiential and bring a whole range of diverse experiences to the forefront. They are possible because we possess the most powerful simulation machines in the world: our brains. These are the portals that allow us to enter these White Spaces and to live realities that are far away in time or physical distance to create possibilities for new possibilities.

An immersion into a White Space was what made it possible

for a group of managers at a nursing home in the Netherlands to build something extraordinary. In the early 1990s, they realized that if their parents developed dementia, they would not want them to end their days at the very institution they were managing. The place was too much like a hospital, without space (pun intended) to care for people and to meet their nonmedical needs. After a year full of exploration and brainstorming sessions, the managers joined forces with a firm of architects and designed what would become a groundbreaking concept. They envisioned, in their White Space, a village in which people with dementia could truly feel comfortable and live the rest of their lives free of stress, enjoyably, and with as much autonomy as possible, while receiving all the care they would need.

The result was Hogewey, which opened in 2009. This facility is a four-acre neighborhood designed like a movie set, in which all aspects of life are replicated realistically. Its 23 houses offer seven different lifestyles reflecting the most common Dutch home environments, all supported by services designed to resemble life in the 1950s. In this "village," 100 percent of the population has a diagnosis of dementia.

The idea was that each of the 152 residents would live out their lives in what the inventors called "normalized small-scale living" conditions. This setting would enable tenants to manage their own households and carry out the activities of everyday life (washing, cooking, shopping) for as long as they could, just as they would in their own homes, but with the aid and encouragement of trained staff. The local pub, for instance, would serve drinks; the supermarket would have aisles full of products that could be taken home; the cinema would show films; the beauty parlor would offer pedicures and manicures; the local clinic would have a physician and a nurse.

What sets this community apart from other types of senior

communities is that the people working in each of these amenities have the necessary training to make the villagers feel comfortable and in control of their own lives for as long as possible without medicalizing them. And not resorting to medication is key. Residents can, for example, go shopping, fill their carts with anything they desire, and take the items home. Once the products are forgotten, they are returned to the shelves, to be part of other shopping experiences. If a resident orders coffee at the restaurant, it is "on the house." When someone's dementia becomes so severe that they are unable to engage proactively in the community, they can take part in sessions where, for instance, they can still enjoy the sights, sounds, and smells of food preparation. Relatives are free to visit at any time. As a result, the need for medication and healthcare interventions has been reduced substantially. Before the village was built, 50 percent of the residents used antipsychotic medications. After they moved to Hogewey, that number decreased to 12 percent. The success of this pioneering initiative provides testimony that care can come with much less reliance on the medical industrial complex and has inspired the construction of similar villages in other countries, each adapted to the local sociocultural context.

While Hogewey was being conceived, built, operated, and replicated, other transformative initiatives were bringing the best knowledge from all the other spaces and incorporating it into the healthcare system. The places where healthcare services are provided and received could be considered Red Spaces.

Red Is the New Rainbow

Of course, the world is still in need of healthcare services. The question is, in what form or context should they be accessed?

The notion that every type of space can contribute to boosting health has resonated throughout the ages. As far back as 500 B.C., the place, or setting, was considered the fourth factor for maintaining or improving health, following the challenge itself, the patient, and the physician. When the few medicines that a doctor had at his disposal were unable to tackle a health problem, the patient would be transferred to a safe, supportive environment where natural or supernatural forces could aid the healing process. Typically, these were temples, such as those devoted to the god Asklepios. These types of surroundings were designed to immerse patients in nature, music, and art in order to restore harmony and promote healing.

This combination of healing ingredients from different spaces motivated the creation of the word "hospital." The word comes from the Latin noun *hospes,* which means both "a guest or visitor" and "one who provides lodging or entertainment for a guest or visitor," and is also the root of "hospice," "hotel," and "hostel." The shift in the sense from a person to various buildings might have happened through the common term *cubiculum hospitalis,* which means "guest-chamber."

Instead of the delightful and soothing guesthouses that they were meant to be, hospitals turned into dark, unhygienic, busy, crowded places that were contributing to higher rates of avoidable deaths. This negative trend led to a correction of their design. At the turn of the 20th century, hospitals were transformed to increase the amount of natural light, airiness, cleanliness, order, and quietness.

This return to the roots of healing was short-lived. With the widespread introduction of anesthesia and antiseptics, hospitals quickly transitioned into settings where new surgical procedures were offered, creating an overcorrection driven by an obsession with sterility. As antibiotics were introduced around the Second

World War and industrialization was becoming the norm, hospitals grew into impersonal behemoths where patients played a passive role and family involvement in care was practically eliminated. As time went by and even more powerful technologies were developed, modern hospitals became something akin to production lines for diagnosing, curing, and treating diseases. Their designs became dreary, featureless, noisy, uninspiring, foreboding, and bleak. This was all part of the overarching mission to fix physical ailments while also containing costs. Was it possible that this advancement in modern technologies, and the buildings in which they were administered, were making us sicker?

Investigations into hospital design have found that poor arrangements of space can harm patients and staff alike through increased levels of anxiety, stress, and mistakes. These realizations have motivated calls to revisit some of the key attributes of the original healing places. Explorations in these spaces have led to the identification of cost-effective ways to incorporate elements of Green Spaces and Blue Spaces into existing and new buildings.

These initiatives have marked the beginning of yet another wave of interest in proving the value of Red Spaces as the best places where true health outcomes can be obtained. These are especially important when a person's level of self-reported health drops into the negative zone because of physical challenges that are best addressed through medical care provided within the walls of an institution.

As this wave of innovation spread around the world, it stimulated the imagination of many diverse groups, one of which was based in a remote part of Colombia. In a village there, the small community hospital was under pressure because of high demand for services and very limited financial resources. Driven by the belief that the essence of innovation is doing more with less, the leaders of the hospital decided to make a few bold moves that would allow them to offer better services to the public at a lower cost. One of the key components of this effort was the re-allocation of 50 percent of the total budget to preventive measures geared toward increasing the levels of health among the population. To achieve this, they renovated the traditional Red Space (what we might understand as the traditional hospital setting) to be more aesthetically appealing, opening views to a large nearby dam and forests. They built a large gym with a climbing wall and opened it to the public 24/7. They created a large kitchen where the community could learn about new approaches to healthy eating. In addition, they trained a large group of community members to visit people in their homes, schools, and workplaces to improve health, increase literacy levels, and encourage healthy daily activities. Equipped with a colorful bus, they traveled to surrounding villages to expand these efforts beyond their borders. To reflect the new vision, the hospital name was changed to La Casa de la Salud (The House of Health). This new name also captured the fact that 80 percent of its activities had shifted to health promotion and disease prevention.

Within a short time, the fruits of this audacious move started to manifest. Child malnutrition in the town was completely eradicated, visits to the emergency room by patients with respiratory conditions who needed oxygen dropped by 90 percent, and a high proportion of beds that were previously occupied by patients with complex chronic diseases remained unoccupied. They were no longer needed by people who had become much better able to adapt to their life challenges in the community.

Halfway around the world, in the central Pacific Ocean, another visionary project was generating new insights about how Red Spaces could improve human health. This initiative, the

North Hawai'i Community Hospital (NHCH), was led by a very successful American entrepreneur and opened in 1996 as a private nonprofit hospital, envisioned to be a different sort of health facility and a place that could illustrate possibilities for the future of medicine. Rather than striving to be "not just another hospital," it aspired to be "the most healing hospital in the world." It combined top Western medical and surgical practices with other healing traditions, offering the best of high tech and high touch. By treating the patient as a whole person (mind, body, and spirit) in the context of family, culture, and community, the hospital itself was seen as a healing instrument. Ninety percent of the rooms were single occupancy. They faced outside, with full-length sliding doors leading to open patios with sitting areas, and were connected by wide hallways. Natural light was prominently featured via skylights throughout the facility, including in operating rooms.

So, what can be learned from these striking examples of reimagined Red Spaces? At the very least, that almost any medical space can be enhanced to improve health. This might be done through interventions as complex as the reconfiguration of the entire layout, or as simple as including houseplants in hospital rooms. Changes like simply adding decorative plants have been found to reduce pain, anxiety, and fatigue and to enhance satisfaction with both the rooms and the care that patients receive.

As a result of an increased appreciation of the positive power of physical spaces on health, Red Spaces are turning into the source of fresh insights and lessons for all other spaces. They are ideal for bringing together many design elements to reduce the TSL and boost health.

As this type of relationship between people and buildings is explored further by professionals in many different industries, the possibilities to reimagine and reinvent the elements of each space and to bring them all together into vibrant new configurations is bound to continue. Entire new disciplines are emerging on the smallest scales. A case in point is neuroarchitecture, which focuses on exploring the psychoneuroimmunological response (the interaction between psychological processes and the nervous and immune systems of the human body) to built environments. This is likely only the beginning.

As scientists continue to dig in to the spaces in which human lives unfold, they will no doubt reveal an increasing number of unexpected and awe-inspiring insights from the huge and constantly growing network of rich connections that surround us.

Simultaneously, you can benefit from bringing insights from each of the spaces into the settings where you work and live—your Violet Spaces. You can reduce the amount of dust and mold in your bedroom or office just by adding houseplants. Offices with plants also can make the entire team feel better about their jobs, reduce their levels of stress, and result in their getting sick less often. Whatever type of greenery you bring into your Violet Spaces, just learning to nurture it may help reduce anxiety, boost attention, and decrease the severity of depression.

As the benefits of multiple spaces converge, it becomes inevitable to recognize that we are all entangled in non-human realms, embedded in rich micro and macro universes daring us to notice many unusual and surprising opportunities to stay healthy.

CHAPTER 7

TRUST YOUR GUT

There it was, support for an idea that appeared insane for half a century. In the year 2000, scientists showed how an invisible microscopic life-form could successfully reproduce inside and manipulate the mind of a mammal. They found that the microbe *Toxoplasma gondii,* or "toxo" for short, could live in rats' brains and hijack them by rearranging connections between the animals' cells. What was the parasite trying to do with this control? It turns out that it was able to convert rats' natural fear of cats into attraction, making them easy prey for their top predator. The benefit to the toxo: to reach cats' guts, the only place on the planet where it can reproduce.

This finding set off alarm bells within the scientific community. Since the 1950s, there had been fears that toxo had the capacity to influence human behavior as well. The results in 2000 showed that such concerns were justified. International evidence indicates that around 30 percent of people in the world are infected by toxo, mostly through the ingestion of soil, water, crop products, or raw food contaminated by cat feces.

This parasite may also be able to trigger changes in people's minds that parallel those in rats'. It has been found, for example, that entrepreneurs are more likely to be infected by toxo than the general population. Undergraduate business majors were shown to be 1.4 times more likely to test positive for this microbe than biology majors. Even further, among business majors those pursuing specialization in entrepreneurship were 1.7 times more likely to test positive than their counterparts studying less risky business subjects. A similar pattern has been found among professionals attending entrepreneurship events. On one occasion, 124 out of 197 attendees (63 percent) were infected by the parasite. Of those, 14 percent had started their own businesses, compared with just 5 percent of the non-infected people who attended the event. Even though it is impossible to prove beyond any doubt that toxo is responsible, the data are compelling.

Similarly, a study in Denmark, based on government tests of pregnant women for toxo, found that those with evidence of the infection were 29 percent more likely to engage in entrepreneurship than those who tested negative. They were 27 percent more likely to found multiple companies and 134 percent more likely to start a venture by themselves. Their businesses were also more successful financially than those of women with negative toxo tests.

The hypothesis is that toxo manipulates people's brains to make them more comfortable quitting their jobs and keener to start their own companies. It may also reflect a reduction in their ability to collaborate with others or to work well as employees. These effects might just as well be explained by the ability of toxo to affect hormone levels (e.g., it increases testosterone) and other neurotransmitters in the human brain (e.g., dopamine, serotonin, and norepinephrine) in ways that favor entrepreneurial efforts.

Although increasing entrepreneurship may sound good or even be welcome, the negative psychological changes induced by toxo could be so serious as to be considered a major public health concern. People with positive tests for the parasite, for example, seem to be more likely to develop a wide variety of mental and neurological conditions. This impact may occur through toxo's effects on genes that control hormonal or immune functions. The conditions that toxo seems to trigger include Alzheimer's disease, obsessive-compulsive disorder, antisocial personality disorder, anxiety disorders, learning disabilities, and, above all, schizophrenia. In fact, it has been estimated that 21 percent of schizophrenia cases in the world are associated with toxo infection. On top of that, toxo infection might make people more likely to refrain from wearing a helmet to protect themselves from head injuries, to swim or drive while intoxicated, and to have suicidal thoughts. It has been estimated that toxo may account for around 17 percent of traffic accidents and 10 percent of suicide attempts worldwide.

The scientific evidence on how a single microbe such as toxo could produce such profound effects across multiple systems and across several species, affecting humanity in so many ways, is just a sliver of a growing body of research. Explorations in this space are revealing many more hidden entities that affect agency and could enhance your capacity to adapt, and hence your ability to stay or become healthy.

A New Organ

Many additional surprises have come from studying all of the microorganisms that live in the human body and their genetic material. Collectively, these are known as the human microbiome. Contrary to popular belief, there is more to it than what lives in your gut. Microbes are also present on your skin and in your eyes, nose, mouth, lungs, genitals, and urinary tract, among most other parts of your body.

By studying these microorganisms, scientists have discovered that an average body includes around 30 trillion human cells and 39 trillion microbial cells. By this measure alone, you are only 43 percent "human." This is generous compared with the proportion viewed through a genomics lens. It is currently estimated that you have 20,000 human genes and 2 million to 20 million microbial genes in your body. According to that estimate, you are only 1 percent human at best.

As is the case with the inhabitants of a borderland between two countries, your microbiome—the aggregate of all bacteria, viruses, fungi, and archaea that coexist very intimately with your own cells—facilitates your interactions with your "outside" environment.

The main contribution of the microbiome to your life is defensive, either as a trainer of your immune system for how to respond to potentially harmful invaders; as part of your armed forces participating in attacks against microorganisms that can cause infections; or as physical and chemical barriers to protect you from disease.

The microbes you carry can also be valuable partners, boosting the functions of the organs they inhabit. Those in your mouth help initiate the digestion of food; create a biofilm to protect the mucosa from physical, chemical, or biological damage; process and deactivate environmental chemicals; and help reduce inflammation. Those in your gut, the largest community of microbes, can harvest energy, especially by breaking down food that your own cells cannot process, such as dietary fiber; increase the absorption of minerals such as iron, magnesium, and calcium; and act as a factory of neurotransmitters, such as serotonin, as well as enzymes, and vitamins that the human component of your body cannot produce on its own, including vitamins K and B_{12}. The yogurt, leafy greens, and other superfoods you eat are like a loving offering to the non-human allies in your body.

Your skin's microbiome contributes to repairing minor damage and enhances your resistance to radiation. The microorganisms found in your urinary and genital systems can enhance or reduce your fertility. Those in your lungs shape the amount and quality of mucus you produce and can even increase the surface area of your lungs capable of absorbing oxygen from the air.

The recognition that most of the cells and genetic material that make up the human body are non-human, and that our ability to adapt and live depends on an unimaginable number of complex and constantly changing conversations with the trillions of creatures in our bodies that outnumber us beginning at birth, bolsters the case that humans should be considered holobionts. This comes from the Greek word *holo,* meaning "whole," and *biont,* meaning unit of life. The term affirms that the idea of human individuality is an oversimplification. In other words, you are more than you might have thought. Instead of an organism made up only of human cells, your body is the host of a much larger, richer, and more intimate ecosystem that includes human cells and cells with different genetic compositions—even from different kingdoms—whose homeostasis and allostasis, and hence health and survival, depend on one another, and cannot be separated from one another.

Inquiries into the human holobiont, with emphasis on what happens within the gut, indicate that the relationship goes much deeper and further, so much so that the non-human component of the holobiont has been regarded as another organ. After all, an organ is any "part of the body that performs a (vital or special) function." This applies to the gut microbiome, without which it would be impossible for you to adapt, responding to the myriad challenges you face every day.

Furthermore, the microbial communities in your gut communicate with your human cells from the time of birth until the very end of life, using the immune system, the neuronal network in the brain, and other chemical languages. The gut microbiome uses these pathways to communicate at a distance with your other vital organs. One of these, known as the gut-brain axis, acts like a subway line via the vagus nerve, allowing two-way messaging between the microbes in the gut at one end and neurons in the hypothalamus—the region that controls emotions—at the other. The same nerve also has stops along the way at the heart and lungs. This dialogue between microbes and neurons, which transcends natural kingdoms, plays a valuable adaptive role by helping you adjust to the constant barrage of challenges that threaten your health from both inside and outside your body.

This is just one of the crucial pathways the gut microbiome uses to communicate with the other vital organs. Another is the liver, which receives all the blood from the intestines and is responsible for breaking down, balancing, and creating nutrients that then get distributed throughout the body. The liver in turn produces bile, which contains many substances, particularly acids and antibodies, which it empties through the gallbladder into the intestines. This path contributes to your health mostly by the combined power of the two organs, the liver and the gut microbiome, to deal with chemical substances by increasing the nutrients that get extracted from the food you eat, by controlling potentially harmful microbes, and by neutralizing toxins that could hurt you. Interestingly, imbalances in the gut microbiome can also affect your kidneys, mostly through chemicals that can lead to kidney stones, renal failure, or poor dialysis.

Lastly, perhaps the richest of the axes is the one connecting the gut microbiome with your lungs, because it involves conversations among citizens of even more kingdoms, as it connects your human, bacterial, and fungal cells, as well as viruses, across the microbiomes and tissues of two organs. The connections between these two microbiomes are likely behind the improvement in asthma that has been observed after surgical operations on the stomach to treat obesity.

An Outlandish Aid

In all of these cases, either through its communication with the intestinal cells or through its connection with the vital organs, the gut microbiome can make optimal contributions to your adaptability. The same is true in the opposite direction. Low microbiome diversity is closely associated with negative levels of self-reported health.

Many activities that are considered quite normal or at least happen frequently in industrialized societies can hinder this superpower and unleash a harmful ripple effect. When a baby skips the birthing canal during a cesarean section, they are deprived of the rich essential foundations of protective bacteria, viruses, and fungi that reside there. Similarly, many aspects of daily life in large North American cities have been shown to weaken these inner allies. Inhabitants of urban regions have gut microbiomes that are less diverse than those of people living in rural areas. This is the result of less exposure to soil, animals, and microbes present in the environment, as well as, above all, greater consumption of ultra-processed foods rich in refined sugar, saturated fats, and animal protein. A westernized diet, in particular, is associated with the loss of beneficial bacteria, the overgrowth of potentially harmful bacteria, and reduced bacterial diversity. These inner conditions lead to genetic and metabolic changes, as well as inflammation, which can trigger a growing number of non-infectious conditions, considered "civilization diseases." The list includes irritable bowel syndrome, celiac disease, colon cancer, obesity, allergies, asthma, cardiovascular disease, bipolar disorder, anxiety disorders, Alzheimer's disease, Parkinson's disease, chronic pain, and stroke. These problems are extremely rare among hunter-gatherers and other in non-westernized populations.

The recognition of the relationship between health, food, lifestyle, and what happens inside the gut has opened the door to the development and use of "functional foods." These enhanced and fortified edible products can be prebiotics (those with nondigestible components such as fiber), probiotics (those that contain live microorganisms), synbiotics (those that include prebiotics and probiotics packaged together), postbiotics (inactivated microbial cells or parts of cells), and nutraceuticals. The purpose of all of these is the same: to augment the adaptive power of your gut microbiome and keep you healthy. These are the more socially acceptable and widely available diet-based options in this space.

In cases where the microbiome is weakened or dysfunctional, causing a disease or not responding to nutritional or medical interventions, a person may require something more drastic (compared with eating some yogurt) to fix it: fecal transplantation. This technique (which could be considered bizarre) is the most extreme approach to restoring the power of the microorganisms in the gut. It involves transferring feces from a person with a healthy microbiome into the intestines of a patient with a compromised microbiome by either enema or capsules.

Is this a completely new idea? No. Fecal transplantation has a long history. It has been used by cultures around the world at least since it was first described in China in the 4th century as a means to control diarrhea and fever. Curiously, many animals follow this practice by eating the feces of peers or other species, using it as a way to increase the diversity of microorganisms in their intestines and help them to digest a greater range of foods.

The scientific foundations for this practice were laid in the 17th century after the invention of the microscope, when it was discovered that stools contain microbes. This was followed by the publication of the first medical book on the therapeutic benefits of feces, in 1696.

After the extensive characterization of multiple bacteria present in the gut in the 20th century, there was a resurgence of interest in fecal transplantation. It arose from the need to control diarrhea caused by the disruption of the gut flora by antibiotics and from the experience of German troops who ate camel feces during World War II (following ancient Bedouin customs) to combat what otherwise would have been fatal dysentery in the desert.

Beginning in the late 1970s, however, it was the negative impact of antibiotics on the gut that most triggered an explosion in research on fecal transplants, with the bacterium *Clostridium difficile* as the main driver. This bacterium can produce a serious inflammation of the colon, which often starts after the infected person has taken antibiotics. It is resistant to treatments and can be lethal. As the most common microbial cause of healthcare-associated infections in US hospitals, it is considered to be an important source of preventable death. Clinical trials studying the effects of fecal transplantation on this infection yielded spectacular results, which led to a renewed interest in this type of intervention.

Up to that point, most of the benefits of fecal transplants

were related to their direct effect on the gut. The really ground-breaking and potentially paradigm-shifting findings emerged early in the 21st century. Studies showed that fecal transplants could change the course of diabetes, curb obesity, and even extend the benefit of cancer treatments from one group of patients to another. Other studies went even further, revealing that fecal transplants have the potential to influence human minds, as they seem to be able to relieve the symptoms of people with depression or anxiety disorders for prolonged periods of time.

From what has been discovered, it is now clear that our ability to adapt and be healthy is a deeply integrated and collaborative effort, so much so that it goes beyond what we might regard as the boundaries of our identity.

Who Are YOU?

Taken together, these insights about the microbiome—just as with toxo infection—are just another nudge toward recognizing the expanding list of invisible forces that are constantly influencing your life. Acknowledging them inevitably adds a new flavor to the notion of *you* as a whole system, especially when you are trying to answer the key questions to rate your own health— How would *you* rate your health: excellent, very good, good, fair, or poor? Why do *you* consider your health to be at that level? What do *you* need to maintain or improve your level of health? Arguably, it is possible that your answers will be heavily influenced by the massive army of microbes that are constantly sending signals to your brain, making self-reported health even more sophisticated as a reflection of your adaptability.

Hypothetically, when you rate your health, you might be coming up with an overall sense of your ability to adapt that has been generated by the trillions of human and non-human cells in your body. So, when somebody reports their health as negative, it is much more than the subjective assessment of an individual human. Instead, it could be an alarm bell warning that the person's whole system is in danger and that something must change immediately to reduce their TSL, prevent unnecessary suffering, and avoid the risk of premature death.

In sum, the microbiome and its close relationship with human cells are opening up new possibilities for adaptation. They invite an appreciation of *you* as much more than a separate, autonomous individual (made exclusively of human cells), who is living in a constantly changing and challenging world. Considering yourself as a holobiont could enable you to make decisions about what you eat that are informed by the growing scientific evidence on the microbiome and functional foods, and on their relationship to your mood, your behavior, and the risk or impact of chronic disease.

These insights challenge the strong sense that you have an unchanging inner self that persists throughout your life. The lessons learned hang a question mark at the end of statements that uphold the idea that you are the master of your own body and that you alone control your interactions with the world around you.

In addition to revealing that most of the genes and cells in your body are non-human, scientists have confirmed that almost all your human cells—except for the neurons and the cells in your eye lenses—will be replaced completely, and many times, during your life. Also, every molecule in your body is made up of particles that have existed for billions of years and that have also been part of the bodies of countless other plants and animals before you.

On the flip side, these findings are unable to override the

feeling that you have been the same distinct individual all your life, able to remember past events as having happened at the center of your own subjective universe. Such a defiant sense of identity is likely to be yet another powerful survival tool, with deep evolutionary and cultural roots.

By feeling strongly that you exist as a separate person, you are more able to control and plan your behavior and to understand the behavior of others.

The illusion of a distinct unit of *you* makes it possible for a multitude of experiences that would otherwise be fragmented to be bound together. It provides a focal point to organize those experiences into coherent stories. These stories then enrich the illusion, for you and others, of a coherent person, and allows you, and those around you, to treat one another as morally responsible beings.

The experience of a distinct and neatly outlined self has advantages from an adaptive perspective because it is what makes it possible for you to think ahead, to make an effort to tackle "external" challenges, to protect your life, and to feel that you can direct it. In short, the illusion is what makes it possible for you to feel healthy.

Nevertheless, the perspective of being deeply entangled with other beings also can be empowering. It provides a bird's-eye view and opens up new possibilities for boosting your ability to adapt in the face of inevitable challenges in highly effective ways, and report positive health.

Both ideas of self can and must coexist. Maybe you have to continue to act as if a distinct self were real—considering yourself a separate, fully human individual. That could be a means of benefiting from what feeling like an independent being brings along, even if you are convinced that it is not the case. It may be much easier than trying to overcome this illusion. Living with false perceptions seems to be part of our daily lives. After all, even though it was proven centuries ago that the sun does not move across the sky, pretty much everyone still talks about "sunsets" and "sunrises."

There are clearly great benefits and insights to be obtained by exploring the elements that influence your health that are so small they are unseen. It is also necessary to pay attention to those factors that are so massive that they, too, become practically invisible. This might be more crucial than ever to your survival as you negotiate the vast network of networks to which you belong.

CHAPTER 8

THE COMPANY YOU KEEP

On April 12, 1945, President Franklin Delano Roosevelt died at the age of 63 from medical ignorance. The brain hemorrhage that killed him was likely caused by extremely high blood pressure, which had remained untreated for at least a decade and had been recorded at the exorbitant level of 300/190 mmHg just an hour before he was pronounced dead.

Roosevelt's death, coupled with the fact that one of every two Americans were expected to die of heart disease at that time, motivated President Harry Truman to sign into law the National Heart Act on June 16, 1948. The law included a seed grant for a 20-year epidemiological heart study. There was such a poor understanding of heart disease then that the initial budget allocated funds to buy ashtrays for staff members.

A few months later, the Framingham Heart Study began. This project, based in Framingham, Massachusetts, extended beyond the initial 20-year period established by the National Heart Act, included multiple generations of the town's inhabitants, and provided important evidence about many issues and connections that were previously unknown. The participants at the outset, regarded as being representative of the US population as a whole, were mostly middle-class factory workers of western European ancestry.

This initiative helped to set "normal values" for many of the indicators of health used by the medical industrial complex. Blood pressure levels, for instance, became acceptable below 120/80 mmHg. The study identified, for the first time, "risk factors" for heart disease, and later stroke and dementia, recognizing that the effects of these health issues are dynamic, varying in degree based on biological, psychological, and social circumstances. As a result, it was possible to confirm that high blood pressure was closely linked to heart attacks and strokes and that it was also associated with cigarette smoking, high cholesterol levels, obesity, and even hormonal changes related to menopause. Such insights led to the creation of a score, which was based on different factors at different levels, to judge a person's overall risk of, say, developing heart disease or having a stroke.

In 2002, the Framingham Heart Study seemed to be running out of steam. It was being superseded by other large-scale population-based projects in the US and other parts of the world. That was the case until a group of external researchers discovered and analyzed a trove of unused paper records from 1970, which contained raw data on the weight of 12,067 participants and on their relationships during the past 32 years. Their analysis revealed that obesity spreads across relationships and social distances as if it were contagious. They found that the likelihood that a person will become obese increases by 57 percent, on average, if one of their friends is obese, and by 71 percent if they are of the same sex.

Thus, even those who feel disconnected may indeed be interconnected. The chances that a person will be obese even appear to increase if their friend's friends' friends are obese, and even if they do not know one another. However, the effect disappears among neighbors who do not regard one another as friends. Furthermore, when any two people consider each other as friends, their likelihood of becoming obese increases by 171 percent!

This kind of initiative highlights the need to uncover the many hidden opportunities to improve human health and longevity by looking at people as members of networks.

Socially Contagious

In general, a human network has two basic elements: people and their connections to one another, also known as relationships, links, or ties. The connections can go in one or two directions. In a family network, for example, the relationship of "father" goes in one direction and that of "daughter" goes in one direction as well. In contrast, the relationship between spouses or between siblings goes in two directions. The same occurs between friends and colleagues. In a workplace setting, the head of a department has a one-directional link with each of their direct reports and vice versa.

The relationships between people within networks tend to generate novel patterns, properties, and behaviors that make the whole more than the sum of its parts. This was illustrated by the social network of participants in the Framingham Heart Study and the way friendship can cause obesity to spread like a virus, across a community.

Your social network can affect your health, both positively and negatively, depending on the number and diversity of the people with whom you are connected. If your network has lots of people, your chances of experiencing positive levels of self-reported health are greater, because your connections give you access to more resources. If many of your connections are health professionals, for example, it could be easier for you to get a second opinion, within days, from a top specialist than it would if you had fewer healthcare connections or none. If many members of your network can offer you social support, you will have an adaptive advantage when you are in need, as they can contribute financially in times of hardship, help with household chores, provide guidance when you need to make critical decisions, and be a source of meaningful emotional support. People with large social networks with these kinds of links, especially those with close family members and friends, are better equipped to maintain positive levels of self-reported health when dealing with mental challenges.

The health effects of social support are even more pronounced within the simplest social networks, namely those involving only two people. It has been consistently found that married people have lower rates of premature death than their unmarried counterparts.

The effect of social support on health can also be negative, however. The clearest example is that of informal caregivers, including children caring for their parents, parents looking after their children, or spouses caring for their partners. These people experience a high prevalence of anxiety, depression, and suicidal ideas. Although their ties are very strong, they typically lack support, are often lonely, frequently rate their health as negative, and have a greater risk of premature death from all causes.

In a subtler way, your health can be affected by the attitudes and behaviors of the closest members of your network. Your likelihood of having started, continued, or stopped drinking alcohol or smoking tobacco as an adult mirrors the choices of your best friends when you were in high school and your parents or siblings at home.

The effects of these clear relationships between your network and your health pale in comparison with those of a powerful and invisible phenomenon that affects you every moment, without you even noticing it. It is called "social contagion."

A network can spread ideas, attitudes, or behaviors from one person to another. In most cases, the person affected cannot sense the influence (intentional or not) of the initiator. This is how fashion and fake news become so powerful.

Celebrities can even change your behaviors. News stories about a celebrity with breast cancer will increase the chances of their fans undergoing screening tests by orders of magnitude over the effect of more general stories about cancer in the media. The same thing can occur with suicide, something that has been documented since the late 18th century, after the publication of *The Sorrows of Young Werther* by Goethe. This has been corroborated by rising numbers of suicides following media coverage of high-profile incidents involving celebrities.

Social contagion can also occur across large geographic areas, like an outbreak of an infectious disease. This was illustrated by the analysis of another unused data set from the Framingham study that focused on the happiness levels of 4,739 people. This overlooked data showed that a person who lives within a mile of a friend and becomes happy increases the probability that the friend will be happy by 25 percent. This figure jumps up to 34 percent for the effect of a happy next-door neighbor.

Companies, another network within many networks, are susceptible to social contagion too. A study looking at a network that included more than 250,000 employees working at 17,000 companies in Denmark, over a period of 12 years, provides an astounding example of this. It found that people hired from an unhealthy organization (one with many people suffering from mental problems) could spread mood, anxiety, and stress-related disorders in their new workplace, especially when they were brought on board as managers.

From all these examples, it is clear that more connectivity can be either highly beneficial or highly detrimental. How is it possible to get more of the former and gain protection from the latter?

The answer may lie within personal social networks.

Opening New Possibilities by Closing Networks

Friendship is so powerful that it has been regarded as "the single most important factor influencing our health, well-being, and happiness." Indeed, the number of friends you had in childhood can predict self-reported health levels in adulthood decades later. Men without friends at a young age are more likely to experience negative levels of self-reported health when they are in their forties. In contrast, having close friendships can reduce your likelihood of developing both mental disorders and physical illnesses, increase your chances of surviving cancer, shorten the time it will take you to recover when you fall sick or have surgery, and even lower your risk of dying prematurely from almost any cause, to a level that could be equivalent to giving up smoking.

Should you, therefore, try to engage a massive number of friends to be a part of your network? This might not be possible. The number of people who can be included in a personal social network is rather limited.

Research on diverse communities, from current hunter-gatherer groups to those that occur mostly in online environments, suggest that a cohesive social network generally includes about 150 people. The members of a network play a major role in increasing access to items and assets that can boost health and in providing psychological support at any given time.

The structure of a social network is typically organized to include people in layers that increase in size as their emotional ties become weaker. The innermost layer includes the most trusted people, such as at least 1 family member, intimate partner, or friend, typically with around 5 people in total. The next layer contains, on average, about 15 close people, including those in the previous layer. From then on, the number in each layer tends to increase in multiples of three, with the strength of the emotional connection continuing to decrease in each layer.

Ordinarily, each person has room for about 15 "best friends," 50 "good friends," and a total of 150 people who could be called just "friends." Beyond this point, there are at least three other layers, consisting of about 500 "acquaintances," 1,500 people whose names can be recalled, and 5,000 recognizable faces.

The word "friend" represents any tie that is co-constructed by two people based on mutual respect, appreciation, intimacy, and liking. Given this definition, "friends" often include members of a person's biological or legally established family and their romantic partners.

People usually spend approximately 40 percent of their social effort—in terms of frequency or duration of interactions—on the 5 members in their closest layer. Twenty percent is allocated to the remaining 10 members of the second layer, which includes those who are close. Thus, 60 percent of one's social time is devoted to just 15 people who are considered "best friends." Who would be on your list?

One of the main barriers to enjoying the adaptive benefits of friendships is that many people experience loneliness as the result of a distressing "generalized lack of satisfying human relationships" and social isolation, even when they are surrounded by other people. A project supported by the British Broadcasting Corporation (BBC) and a free museum and library called the Wellcome Collection has shed some light on this phenomenon. Based on data collected online from 46,054 participants aged 16 to 99 and living across 237 countries, islands, and territories, the study found that loneliness increases with individualism, decreases with age, and occurs more frequently in men than in women. It is surprising to note that the stereotype of being socially isolated does not belong to older people, but instead can be assigned to another group. Disturbingly, the most vulnerable group is younger men (between the ages of 14 and 24) living in individualistic cultures. Forty percent of them said they felt lonely, compared with 27 percent of those over 75. The numbers in the US, in particular, are staggering, with a survey of 10,000 adults conducted in 2019 finding that 61 percent of adults said they experienced loneliness, an increase of 7 percent compared with the previous year.

The prevalence of loneliness, which seems to be increasing around the world, is considered a public health concern, mainly because of overwhelming evidence about the deleterious effects that it can have on health. Loneliness makes people more prone to having two or more diseases and significantly increases the risk of dying early of almost any cause. A lonely person faces an increased risk of heart attack, stroke, Alzheimer's disease, obesity, poor sleep quality, diabetes, anxiety, depressed mood, addiction, and suicidal ideas. In fact, analysis of data from more than 3.4 million people found that loneliness is associated with a 26 percent increase in the risk of an earlier death, equivalent to the effect of smoking 15 cigarettes a day. What adds to the concern about this issue is the finding that loneliness is socially contagious and is resistant to the protective effects of income, education level, sex, and ethnicity.

Even though many interventions have been proposed to reduce loneliness and its effects on health, they typically focus on confronting the issue of social isolation through "direct" approaches. These include "befriending" calls by volunteers; "social skills training" courses; and even robots to eliminate the need for human-to-human interaction. In addition, lonely people are often targeted "indirectly" through activities that make interactions with others inevitable (e.g., group exercise programs), and even through psychotherapy to modify biased perceptions of and negative tendencies toward interacting comfortably with others.

These interventions tend to focus on older people rather than the younger groups who are more strongly impacted by social isolation. A key problem with these options is that they operate on a third-person basis, considering the lonely person as a customer, client, or patient who would benefit from being "inserted" into a network of "services" with "fixes" for them. Unsurprisingly, their effects at the personal and societal levels are either modest or mixed at best. The interest in using robots to eliminate the need for human-to-human interaction as a modern approach to addressing loneliness is just an extreme variation on the same artificial and impersonal theme.

The Power of "Withness"

Given that loneliness has become yet another item on the growing list of existential threats, it is time to consider an alternative approach to it, one that is tried-and-true and has existed since time immemorial. We like to call it "proactive social networking," which incorporates many of the elements found in strong traditional tribes. In essence, proactive social networks are groups of people who align their interests to boost adaptability.

As the name indicates, these kinds of social networks are created for a reason. This could be to pursue a common higher purpose, vision, or mission that strengthens the ties among members. They might focus on political action, such as being part of the anti-war movement in the US during the 1960s and '70s, the protests against the World Trade Organization in the late 1990s, or Extinction Rebellion, a movement aimed at averting the collapse of civilization because of human-driven climate change and ecological breakdown. Because of this kind of focused energy, proactive social networks create the opportunity for loosely linked networks to overlap. This allows members from various groups to participate in multiple social networks or expand and reconfigure existing ones. Other proactive social networks could be created around a hobby, sport, or creative endeavor.

Perhaps the most (apparently) easy-to-assemble proactive social network is what could be called a "family by choice." This term refers to a network, with roots in prehistoric human clans, in which each person is linked to others by ties that are equivalent to those of a biological family. In a family by choice, people designate one another as relatives, usually to fill gaps created by geographic or emotional distance from their biological families. In this way, it is possible to complement a biological family or to overcome loneliness and social isolation resulting from other causes such as social intolerance. A "created" or "chosen" family helps members to achieve levels of physical, emotional, and social support and safety that are rarely found in any other type of human grouping.

For a proactive social network to become sturdy and dependable, it must have one indispensable ingredient: trust. Trust is viewed as a social emotion because it is only possible *with* others, and because only with trust is it feasible for very large populations to enjoy positive health and adaptability. This is demonstrated by the best healthcare system in the world, built in Latin America on a shoestring with a trusted network as its foundation.

Proactive networks come with yet another built-in ingredient, which is often underappreciated, because most of the attention is placed on the people who are its members. That ingredient is the rich set of connections that link the people in your life. It is said that "music is created by the spaces between the notes." Similarly, adaptability occurs between the nodes (the people) and across the connections of a social network.

These connections can be described as, or brought to life by, verbs. "To trust" is a prominent option, which in turn includes "to believe," "to serve," and "to support." Other frequent alternatives are "to listen," "to understand," "to share," and "to explore."

The word "connection" itself includes an important clue as to how to get the most out of the networks to which you belong. The verb "connect" comes from the Latin *conectere*, meaning "to join together." It captures an essential aspect of health and adaptability in general: Both are experienced with others.

It is impossible to be healthy or to adapt to the future alone. It is not "I" or "you" or "he" or "she" who can be healthy or adapt; it is always "we." We can only be healthy and adapt with one another. Together.

Expanding Your Connections

The boundaries of your own effective personal social network, with its limited number of people in each layer, can be expanded to boost your ability to adapt. The trick lies in mobilizing your existing tight bonds, not building new relationships. For example, imagine that you are struggling to adapt, and the challenge you face is beyond the ability of your 15 best friends (those people in your innermost layer) to support you. What if you called on one of them to activate a member of their own group of 15 to help you? Given that the bond is so tight between you and your friend, and between your friend and their friend, you would not need to build a new separate connection with the latter (which would dilute the strength of the links in your network, making it less effective). You could gain adaptability from the link between your friend and their friend while still keeping your network intact. In other words, you could benefit indirectly from another trustworthy person without having to join each other's networks. Likewise, that person, or any other person related to them, could benefit just as much from you or other members of your closest layer. Thus, your individual and collective potential to adapt can be supercharged by the high levels of trust, commitment, and generosity embedded in a practically endless chain of intentional "networks of networks."

The capacity to supercharge personal social networks increased in the first two decades of the 21st century thanks to the widespread penetration of digital telecommunication tools. Now, practically everyone can be of support to, and be supported by, anyone else around the world. In theory, this level of access to the whole human network should give you an unprecedented capacity to adapt to almost any existing or new challenge. As a result, your network of networks could even play a key role in tackling some of the biggest challenges to health. The connection between health and climate change is a clear case in point. After all, the climate crisis is responsible for causing increased risks of cancer, infection, respiratory and heart problems, diabetes, birth defects, impaired sleep, anxiety, and suicide, all of which bring with them greater utilization of healthcare services, costs, and premature mortality.

To raise the stakes even further, in 2020, the WHO declared climate change and air pollution together as the biggest threat to global health in the 21st century. At that point, diseases caused by pollution—mostly of air, water, and soil—were responsible for 16 percent of all human deaths worldwide. That was 3 times the number of deaths from AIDS, tuberculosis, and malaria combined, and 15 times the number caused by all wars and other forms of violence on the planet. Furthermore, more than 70 percent of deaths and diseases associated with pollution occurred in low- and middle-income countries.

In light of what we know about the power of human social networks and massive challenges like this one and others that will occur, the key questions become: Why are we not mobilizing the power of cooperation, solidarity, and collective ingenuity to the best of our abilities? Why do we continue to hamper our own individual and collective ability to adapt?

The answer may lie in the way in which we evolved. Choosing clear paths to survive and thrive appears to be much harder than expected.

CHAPTER 9

GETTING OUT OF YOUR OWN WAY

What makes you uniquely human?

This is a question we have asked at conferences and large gatherings of people when exploring the essential questions of our time. Usually when we put it out there as a topic of discussion, some people immediately say, "Art!" We then show them how robots driven by artificial intelligence can produce paintings and music that are practically indistinguishable from world-class human-made art. Others propose altruism, compassion, empathy, or the capacity to experience love, only to be shocked by evidence suggesting that these are likely present in the animal world too.

As we have explored this question further, the list of possibilities has gotten shorter and shorter. We have found that even something so quintessentially associated with humanity as farming and domesticating animals at the same time is not unique to people. Longfin damselfish have domesticated a kind of shrimp to help them grow the algae they eat. The thick-footed morel, a mushroom, does something similar. It cultivates the bacteria that live within its networks, essentially planting bacterial populations there, then harvesting and consuming them. In addition, we are not the only ones with intuitive abilities—the capacity to remember, to imitate, to reason, to be curious, to guess the state of mind of others, or to feel empathy or compassion. Other animals have them too.

We are not even the only ones who are self-aware. What other living being can possibly do this? There is evidence confirming that the great apes, as well as elephants, dolphins, and even birds such as the European magpie, are able to recognize themselves. This evidence has motivated governments around the world to start giving animals non-human person rights.

One by one, the answers offered to the question of what makes us unique have been rebutted. We humans used to view ourselves as the only creatures with morality, politics, and culture, or the only ones who have a sense of fairness or are able to use money or cook. Not anymore.

Even our darkest qualities are shared. Other animals can also be envious, jealous, manipulative, and deceitful. They can get drunk or bully, rape, kidnap, or kill others for trivial reasons. They can also wage war.

Our uniqueness is being challenged by nonliving beings as well. Increasingly, machines are showing that they can be just as good as people at performing tasks that require high levels of creativity. Besides being able to compose music and create paintings comparable to those of top human artists, they are even better at deploying highly specialized skills, such as those involved in diagnosing diseases, performing surgery, and making financial decisions. We have already created machines that can communicate in their own languages, beyond our comprehension; that are learning to cooperate using rules too complex for us to grasp; and that can even ask questions formulated by themselves. This is why the path to non-human personhood is opening up for artificial beings too.

So, what is unique to us, as humans?

What if it is our ability to make bad decisions, even knowing that the outcomes will be unfavorable—our predilection for self-harm and self-destruction?

We may be the only creatures that lay our own traps, are lured by them, and get caught in them.

There seems to be something underlying our intention and our will that warps how we act so that we go against our better judgment and bear the negative consequences that we, in many cases, could anticipate. We like to call this stubborn enigma that fuels irrationality the Self-Destructive Force.

Negatives Attract

As is the case with the toxic stress load, nobody seems immune to this force.

At any given point, in the US alone, 72 percent of adults report having at least one unhealthy behavior or avoidable risk factor, including insufficient sleep, obesity, physical inactivity, smoking, or excessive drinking. All of these are closely related to increased rates of chronic disease and premature death. The odds of reporting negative health double for those with one unhealthy behavior.

Could it be that people do not know any better? No. Lack of knowledge is not the problem, as these behaviors and risk factors tend to match the items most frequently found at the top of the lists of resolutions that people around the world make at the beginning of each year. Their high failure rate is also similar worldwide. By the second week of February, 80 percent of people have failed to meet their resolutions, with only about 8 percent succeeding by the end of the year.

The tendency to do something potentially harmful, even when knowing the likely outcome, also manifests in other physically self-destructive behaviors that are highly prevalent in every society around the world. These include self-injury—such as cutting, hair pulling, scratching, hitting, or burning—which is present in up to half of adolescents, more than one-third of university students, and a quarter of adults.

Self-inflicted harm is not always physical. It can also be psychological, which tends to have mostly social consequences. At the top of the list is self-sabotage, also called self-handicapping. This happens when you put obstacles in your own way, along a path that is meant to bring benefits to you. It is captured by expressions like "shooting yourself in the foot" or "voting against your own interests." In other words, self-sabotage involves foolish behavior that requires your complicity in creating misery for yourself, especially when everything seems to be going well for you.

The most frequent way to accomplish this derailment is by procrastinating. Instead of acting when you are facing an opportunity to do well, you make excuses to justify your inaction, causing unnecessary and potentially harmful delays. Other frequent forms of self-sabotage are comfort eating, particularly when you have a weight loss objective; going to bed late and waking up tired before an important exam or meeting; failing to train before a key event; picking a fight with a loved one when things are going smoothly; and engaging in a physical activity that results in an injury the day before a major competition.

A close variation on self-sabotage or self-handicapping is the impostor syndrome—the persistent sense of self-doubt about your own abilities and merits. This is most common among high-achieving individuals who doubt the reasons for their accomplishments and dread being exposed as a fraud. This often leads them to aggressive efforts to achieve even more, while not being able to accept recognition when they have clear successes. This results in increased levels of anxiety, stress, and burnout, which end up hindering their overall performance. Depending on the tests used to detect impostor syndrome, it affects up to 82 percent of people in positions of responsibility, such as physicians, nurses, managers, and teachers. Women seem to experience it more often than men, and in both sexes the frequency decreases as the person ages.

Self-destructive behaviors can also take the form of compulsive activities—repetitive behaviors that have negative consequences. At the top of the list by far—surpassing drug use, gambling, gaming, hoarding, compulsive sex, and internet use—is compulsive buying and binge eating. These forms of harmful behavior affect huge swaths of the US population, with one-third reporting over-shopping and 50 percent binge eating.

Additionally, it is possible to inflict harm on yourself through impulsive and risky activities that have physical consequences. It is estimated that 75 percent of Americans aged 15 to 44 have unprotected sex with sporadic partners or even with people they just met, and that half of the deaths resulting from car crashes happen when people are not wearing seatbelts.

The ultimate form of self-harm is suicide, which is responsible for more deaths around the world than either AIDS, malaria, breast cancer, war, or homicide. Most suicides occur in people before the age of 50, with men dying by suicide 2.3 times more frequently than women across the globe.

This drive for what is detrimental is fed by what is known as "negativity bias," the human propensity to pay more attention to and react to the most unfavorable, unpleasant, or traumatic situations or events, rather than to the most convenient, pleasant, or soothing ones. Thus, losing money, being abandoned or hurt by family or friends, and receiving criticism usually have a greater and longer-lasting impact on you than their positive counterparts. These kinds of negative experiences generally affect you more than winning money, being accompanied and loved by friends and family, and receiving praise. This means that a single traumatic experience can throw you into a tailspin, with long-term effects on health, well-being, attitudes, self-esteem, anxiety, and behavior. In contrast, there is little evidence that a single positive experience can have an equally consequential upside.

This pervasive mental focus on the negative makes you more vulnerable to experiencing poor health and getting stuck in a downward spiral rife with opportunities to add to your TSL. It also makes you less able to adapt to challenges and less motivated to engage in constructive behaviors and attitudes. This selectively targeted attention on the negative makes bad health have a greater impact on happiness than good health, and pessimism a stronger influence on your health than optimism. Generally speaking, bad is stronger than good.

Inner Sources

What is fueling the Self-Destructive Force? Our strong tendency to hurt ourselves, at all levels, from the individual to the species, might result from an adaptive response turned maladaptive.

Negativity bias is thought to have been advantageous in evolutionary terms. Organisms that were better attuned to potentially harmful events were more likely to survive threats and had increased chances of passing along their genes. The same goes for humans. Our quintessential hunter-gatherer ancestors who misinterpreted the cause of a rustling bush near a watering hole as something trivial, even once, may have ended up handicapped or dead. In contrast, those who overlooked a positive opportunity may have felt some regret but would not have been hurt directly as a result. Therefore, it is adaptively more profitable to be ready to respond more strongly to something negative than to something positive.

This archaic mechanism, which tends to focus your attention on the negative, can turn into a disadvantage, especially when it inhibits your ability to latch on to, cherish, and get a boost from the positive. In essence, when negativity bias becomes maladaptive, it makes you naturally devalue and avoid goodness, and even perceive it as a source of weakness.

The attraction to the negative is also reflected in our culture, fueling the Self-Destructive Force. Essentially, you become what you see or consume. To a degree, you end up imitating the stories that move you. Since positive news, movies, and novels about happy relationships, and perfect lives in general, are rarely commercial successes, you are surrounded by darker plots. Far from being driven by the malicious intent of outside creators, the Self-Destructive Force is fueled by your built-in negativity bias and the hand of the market.

Simply put, terrible information seizes our attention and receives more conscious processing, making bad news and distressing dramas more effective at reaching or engaging wider audiences. This in turn stimulates the creation of even more negative content, which people continue to imitate in progressively more self-destructive ways, multiplying the downfalls and bad decisions of their attractive characters. Ultimately, this creates an environment in which dysfunctional lives are just "the way life is."

The negativity bias fueling the Self-Destructive Force can also feed the social urge to be different. Being good tends to be perceived as dull, unoriginal, or even something that should be punishable. In contrast, naughty or destructive alternatives tend to be perceived as more attractive and effective ways of standing out. This thirst for notoriety could propel, at least in part, the growing prevalence of risky, self-damaging behaviors on a large scale.

Along the same lines, a modern culture that rewards strong, individualistic people with high self-esteem can easily become a hotbed of this force. This is especially true in an environment in which the self, and in particular a person's sense of worth and image, are dependent on variable and fragile circumstances that are out of their hands. Thus, some people go so far as to hurt their chances of success deliberately, as a way to avoid taking responsibility for their failures, thus protecting their identity. In other words, self-handicapping allows a person to find an external source to blame for potential failures, even if doing so ends up having a significantly negative impact on their success, as long as it protects their ego. This strategy can be seen among athletes who create disastrous situations in their personal lives at the peak of their professional careers. If they are unable to perform optimally, they have concocted a set of excuses for their failure, which are not a reflection of their skills. In this way, the ultimate goal is achieved. Their self-esteem is safe.

The Self-Destructive Force can also originate from a different default that is constantly at play: your inability to perceive time, and yourself through time, and to develop a "connection" with your future self. This relationship, even though it seems like it would be an intimate one, can often feel more like a weak bond, especially when the distance in time is great. Your future self may seem like a completely different person altogether, like a stranger. To illustrate this, imagine your next birthday. What will the celebrations look like? Can you imagine yourself in this scene? Now do the same for your birthday in 10 years. The connection you feel to your future self a decade into the future will likely be much weaker than the connection to the self you envisioned a year from now.

The degree of closeness between your present and future selves can influence your health and well-being. It has been found that the strength of the connection people feel to their future selves shapes whether they will act in such a way as to ensure their well-being down the line. People who have a stronger bond through time tend to accumulate more assets, choose more ethical (rather than unethical) courses of action, exercise more, and procrastinate less.

Self-destructive behavior can be connected with the past as well, particularly with traumatic events early in life (often caused by someone else's manifestation of this force). Children who were exposed to highly negative situations have twice the risk of inflicting self-harm as adults. Traumatic events include sexual or other forms of abuse, emotional neglect, divorce or separation of parents, and parents suffering from mental illness or spending time in jail. This is the situation for around 40 percent of children, on average, worldwide, as well as for half of the children in the UK and 60 percent of those in the US.

Research has shown, consistently, that children who experience major negative events are more likely to smoke cigarettes, have problems with alcohol, use illicit drugs, and engage in risky sexual behavior later in life. Furthermore, the lifelong economic impact of childhood trauma might be bigger than that of all other major pediatric health problems, including autism, asthma, cancer, exposure to environmental pollution, and obesity. In addition, the impacts of trauma can be transmitted to the next generation and can even result from genetic changes in the mothers' eggs, which are triggered by their own traumatic experiences as children.

Something as frequent as a child's being separated from one or both parents—which 40 to 50 percent of children in the US experience—can lead to a significant increase in the risk of suicide attempts and self-harm during their late teens and young adulthood. Those separated from their father at birth have more than double the risk, and those separated from both parents have an increase of five to six times the risk, as compared with those living with both parents. The impact of separation from parents on the mental health of children in general seems to be greater than the effect of parental death.

Another theoretical source of the Self-Destructive Force comes from the world of psychoanalysis and is much harder to prove: the death drive, the unconscious tendency that people have to revert to their original inorganic state by ceasing all of their functions and eliminating all of their causes of tension.

Other theories to explain this appetite for self-destruction go beyond the individual mind and zoom out to the species level. How is that even possible?

Overwhelming Powers

In theory, the Self-Destructive Force could be driven by non-human mind manipulators. Although this may sound like science fiction, take this scene as an example: A worker ant is going about the forest ground looking for resources for its colony, and along the way it happens to come into contact with a special kind of fungal spore. Nothing seems to change. The ant continues about its business. This seems like something that can easily be ignored. However, the contrary is brutally true. The spore has stuck to the ant's body and slipped a fungal cell inside it. The cell begins to multiply until the fungus makes up nearly half of the ant's body mass. Once it reaches a certain point, the fungus, called *Ophiocordyceps unilateralis,* takes over the ant's body by infiltrating its muscles and sending chemicals to its brain to execute the fungus's own final stage of development. The fungus drives the ant to leave its colony and quickly climb the nearest plant. Once it gets high enough, the ant bites into the stem or trunk, locks its jaws, and dies. Out of the ant's head, a giant stalk bursts forth and releases a downpour of spores onto the ant trails below. This is yet another dramatic case of cross-species mind manipulation.

Fungi have no hands or mouths to manipulate the world, but they have been regarded as powerful messengers throughout history. Ayahuasca, magic mushrooms, peyote, and other entheogens (psychedelic substances) have been used by shamans and other priestly figures in most cultures around the world as non-human life-form that can borrow the human body and use the brain and senses to communicate with us.

These striking examples may be at the extreme of a spectrum, highlighting the hypothetical possibility that tiny biological entities could be hijacking our mental functions. Some could be active on a very large scale, allowing individuals to feel that they are functioning pretty normally while manipulating them to engage in acts of mass self-destruction, as in the case of toxo.

Given that there is still a lot to be learned, it is reasonable to ask: What could be "wearing us"? Maybe the Self-Destructive Force is the manifestation of a fungus or a prion (a pathogenic protein). Who knows, it could be how the earth is defending itself against us from all the harm we have caused, trying to get rid of us by turning us against our very selves. It could also be part of the survival strategy of communities of microbes vying for a return to the world dominance they enjoyed for billions of years.

Maybe this force is part of the second law of thermodynamics, a manifestation of entropy, pushing us toward chaos and destruction. It could be that resisting it is not only impossible as individuals and as a society, but simply part of a natural law.

Although more options to explain our self-destructive urges will likely continue to emerge, at some point we will start pushing up against the unknowable. Countless scientists, philosophers, religious leaders, mystics, and artists throughout the ages have recognized that there are realities that escape our grasp; there are limits to our rationality and logic to discover what is "out there" as well as within. For starters, what we perceive to be real is anything but. We are incapable of seeing reality as it is because that is not helpful to us, at least not from an evolutionary standpoint. Maybe the Self-Destructive Force is just as far out of the reach of our understanding as some other major issues, such as what happens after we die.

Even though there are many possibilities that could explain the source of this force, the main message from existing views about how to reduce its impact is the age-old evolutionary dictum: Only the fittest—those with the greatest ability to adapt—will survive.

Beyond Willpower

How can you adapt and be healthy under the influence of the Self-Destructive Force? The message from research is clear: Willpower alone is not enough.

Please note that if your TSL is overwhelming, it is essential to seek professional support. This is particularly relevant if you are experiencing suicidal ideas, if you feel that you have a habit that is out of control, or if someone close to you has expressed concern about a behavior of yours that they think is compulsive or potentially dangerous. In addition, if you are engaging in any other self-destructive behaviors and your levels of self-reported health have become negative (that is, you rate your health as poor or fair) or are declining quickly (e.g., from excellent to good in a matter of hours or days), you, too, might benefit from reaching out to a professional.

Through our work around the world with various populations of different cultures, we have identified an antidote of sorts that can enhance your ability to adapt to challenges that are self-created, regardless of how seriously self-destructive the behaviors might be. We have concluded that the core requisite of all forms of protection against this force is recognizing that facing it alone is futile.

You will always require companionship and backing from close people in your life who are willing to work with you as you combat the Self-Destructive Force. One way to achieve this is by building what we call a "personal board of directors."

Just like a corporate board of directors, created to provide guidance and oversight to encourage prosperity within an organization, your personal board acts like a team of confidants to advise you and give you feedback on your life decisions. They can also guide you while you identify and tackle the inevitable challenges you will encounter while fighting the urge to hurt yourself.

It is possible to curate your personal board of directors and design how it will work and how it will support you. The key is for the board to be a joyful addition to your healthy life, rather than a burden contributing to negative health or reinforcing your self-destructive tendencies.

Enlisting someone as a member of your board is a serious endeavor and should be approached with prudence. There are two questions you should ask yourself when considering whom to engage: Whom can you truly trust? Who really has your best interests in mind, even when you are in self-destructive mode? The people identified through these questions tend to be the best ones to keep close, especially when you least want to hear what they have to say.

Once you have this group assembled, you can even use negativity bias in your favor to counteract the power of the Self-Destructive Force. Since the power of the dread of loss and failure is stronger than the attraction of gain or the achievement of success, you can channel this energy toward beneficial outcomes through the creation of challenges with members of your board. For instance, you might make a bet with them, a wager of sorts, aimed at avoiding unhealthy weight gain or lack of exercise. In essence, as someone with a board of directors or as a member of someone else's board, the objective is to turn harmful choices into the hardest ones to make, thus paving the way for more beneficial alternatives to materialize.

Together, as you gain experience protecting one another, you may notice that a frequent manifestation of the Self-Destructive Force is insatiability. You may find yourselves on a never-ending treadmill of wants and needs. This is completely natural. You are living evidence of how successful the species has been at outcompeting all others. The biggest challenge now is to understand that the art of living well lies in striking the right balance between having too much and really needing so little.

The central question now becomes: How much is enough?

CHAPTER 10

WHEN IS ENOUGH ENOUGH?

Since the industrial revolution, there has been a flare-up of an old human ailment that is highly contagious and distressing and that has remained widely unchecked: overconsumption and its consequences, also known as "affluenza."

Affluenza is a socially transmitted condition that results "from the dogged pursuit of more." Its manifestations are clear in the US, the most afflicted country in the world. From 1986 to 2021, for instance, the nation's consumer spending consistently made up more than 60 percent of GDP, trending toward 70 percent year over year.

Could this pattern of extreme consumption be driven by a need to fulfill a significant lack? This is hardly the case. Americans represent 4 percent of the world's population and yet occupy 90 percent of the total space on the globe dedicated to self-storage. This detrimental condition is seen across all generations, not just adults with credit cards. American children, who represent 3 percent of the world's total child population, consume 40 percent of all the toys produced on the planet.

Although affluenza is an affliction driven by those in the wealthiest countries, it has spread throughout the world, impacting people at all income levels. Those at the bottom are stricken twice, since they are conditioned to want an opulent lifestyle but have few possibilities of attaining it. Some of the restrictions on fulfilling these aspirations are natural, as it is physically impossible for every person in the world to consume as much as the average person in a high-income country. Humans would need 3.8 earths to sustain this lifestyle for all. In contrast, if everyone's consumption matched the levels of the average person in the world, humanity would sit right at the level of sustainability and would even have a little breathing room.

This challenge is one that we have to face as a species. We essentially live in the digestive tract of a massive machine, surrounded by things that have already been consumed or by neatly packaged items ready to be used and turned into waste.

In any case, affluenza has created a culture that characterizes success with words such as "bigger," "better," "faster," and "greater." We are destined to fail because our desires are unlimited. We are, in fact, insatiable.

How does this affect your health or your ability to adapt? In prehistoric times, as groups of humans went through times of scarcity, a tendency to accumulate more food and nonfood items than needed was protective (to be stored for times of scarcity). Those who indulged were sending messages of fitness to potential mates and of a high capacity to protect others in the group as well as their own future offspring. This excess, however, came at a risk to our ancestors. Those carrying extra items could be spotted more easily by predators and rivals, and the items would make it more difficult for them to escape. In a way, we are the descendants of the hoarders who survived.

During the times of abundance that we are experiencing now, excess also comes at a cost, albeit a quite different one. Beyond the fact that overconsumption has devastating effects on the biosphere (think air pollution and chemicals in our water), which hurt you indirectly, insatiability can be directly fatal when you interact with the medical industrial complex. This space could hardly be considered a safe zone. Instead, it is full of deadly traps inside and around its perimeter. When it comes to medicine, an excess or a lack could cost you your life. Given that it is so easy to miss the mark, it is vital to ask: What is enough?

Too Much Medicine

There is a fine line between doing too little and doing too much. Sometimes doing nothing carries risk, including not using an effective vaccine, not performing a particular test, or waiting for some symptom to go away. Even staying in bed "resting" can cause lethal blood clots in the legs. More common, though, are the harms associated with doing too much.

Given our evolutionary history, it is natural and in principle good for your adaptability to worry and be alert about potential risks. At a time of abundant medical resources, more might seem like a good idea and soothe your worries in the present. However, more medicine, by itself, may become a greater risk than what was worrying you in the first place.

There is such a thing as "too much medicine." This happens when diagnoses or medical activities increase with very little gain. More is done with lesser results, and in many cases causes much more harm than good.

What is underlying this excessiveness? Everyone is trying to protect themselves: patients, doctors, insurers, sales representatives, researchers, politicians, investors, administrators, and the list goes on.

Too much medicine is manifested through expanded disease definitions, the invention of bogus illnesses, uncritical adoption of population screening, commercial vested interests, intransigent clinical beliefs, increased patient expectations, litigation, aversion to uncertainty, and the unnecessary introduction of new technology. All of this stokes your natural urges as an individual to do more, making you feel that you are contributing to your adaptability. Instead, your efforts may be pushing you into harm's way by increasing the number of unnecessary encounters with the medical industrial complex. This is seen all over the world, with doctor visits ranging from an average of 2 per person per year in Costa Rica to more than 17 in South Korea.

What is the best way to avoid harm from medical overconsumption? There are opportunities to curb this negative outcome by managing anxiety and better judging what is enough in terms of worrying, testing, diagnosing, treating, informing, and improving.

TAMING FEAR OF DISEASE

General population data indicate that 3 to 13 percent of people are hypochondriacs. These are people who display exaggerated anxiety and preoccupation because of the belief that they have a serious disease, based on the misinterpretation of bodily symptoms, in the absence of known diseases, and despite appropriate medical evaluation and reassurance. At the root, hypochondriasis is an adaptive mechanism—to be concerned about your own health and survival—that has become maladaptive. The number of people who are hypochondriacs is quite high in specialist clinics, where one out of five people fit this description. In psychiatric practices, the number is one out of three.

In many cases, hypochondriasis appears when a relative or

close friend becomes seriously ill or dies, or after recovering from a potentially lethal disease. It has been stigmatized and deemed largely to be an imaginary condition. Hypochondriasis is often described in terms of "health anxiety," even though some professionals believe that these are two separate and frequently overlapping problems.

It has also been shown that patients with severe health anxiety use healthcare services 40 to 80 percent more than the general public. Likely because of an elevated toxic stress load, these patients have a 70 percent increased risk of heart disease and a 47 percent increase in the odds of dying prematurely from any cause.

What is the best way to deal with this type of excessive fear or worry? The first thing is to remember that you are far from alone. Many people worry a lot about their own health, or the risk of missing something serious by not paying enough attention to concerning signals. You are likely worrying too much when you continue to doubt several negative test results or the comments made by doctors who calmly tell you that everything seems fine. As a treatment for excessive worry, or hypochondriasis, it is preferable to try non-pharmacological therapies first to reduce the chances of avoidable harm associated with adverse drug effects. Cognitive behavioral therapy, either in person or virtually administered, seems to relieve 66 percent of cases and leads to remission 48 percent of the time.

CURBING OVERTESTING

Too much medicine usually begins when clinicians request and perform tests that are unlikely to yield useful findings. Why does this happen? There are multiple reasons. Overtesting is often the result of fear of accusations of malpractice and litigation, pressure from patients, a culture that promotes a "more is better" attitude and behaviors, or perverse financial incentives. Sometimes, it can even result from laziness or convenience, as strange as that may sound. Usually it is easier for a physician to order a test than not to.

Ordering unnecessary tests can lead to preventable harm because it increases the chances of getting false positives, which can incorrectly suggest that there is something wrong. This could then trigger a cascade of additional investigations and tests to clarify the situation, which can add to the TSL by needlessly scaring a patient and their loved ones. Overtesting also consumes finite resources that could be used more beneficially for other cases.

It has been estimated that in primary care, urine cultures to identify bacteria are overused up to 77 percent of the time in the US, 50 percent in Sweden, and 36 percent in Spain. Family physicians have been shown to be seven times more likely than specialists to request repeat blood tests. In emergency rooms, 85 percent of physicians acknowledge that they order unnecessary tests as part of the "wide nets" they cast to avoid missing important diagnoses. Elsewhere in hospitals, it has been observed that 60 to 70 percent of laboratory tests "are potentially inappropriate or of doubtful clinical importance."

Overtesting also occurs frequently when non-recommended tests are used to try to catch undiagnosed diseases in asymptomatic patients. This is the case with "checkups"—also known as "general medical exams," "periodic health evaluations," or "wellness visits"—which aim at identifying and preventing diseases in people who feel otherwise healthy and who have easy access to healthcare services. A careful analysis of 31 studies with follow-up from 1 to 30 years concluded that annual checkups, and all of their associated tests, fail to reduce premature mortality and are also ineffective in lowering the risk of cardiovascular disease or cancer.

CONTAINING OVERDIAGNOSIS

On many occasions, preventable harm happens when someone who is asymptomatic is given the label of a pathological condition on the basis of abnormalities that sound worse than they really are, when in reality they are not destined to ever bother the person or "will never cause symptoms or death."

When does overdiagnosis mostly happen? There are many instances. It occurs when screening programs result in the detection of lesions that will never grow or never become a problem. This often happens with mammograms, or when imaging technologies, such as total body scans as part of an annual checkup, identify tiny "abnormalities" that will forever remain benign.

Overdiagnosis also happens because of how diseases are defined. You might think that medical doctors use fixed criteria to determine whether and when someone has a condition, such as diabetes or even cancer. Far from it. In reality, professional medical associations with task forces or committees decide the levels at which diseases should be regarded as present or absent. These criteria can change depending on their decisions. When they do, it can have widespread consequences, often labeling generally healthy people as sick. In the US, a lowering of the threshold for normal blood pressure in 2017 increased the proportion of adults diagnosed with hypertension from around one-third to almost one-half of the entire adult population.

Even more broadly, overdiagnosis occurs through the medicalization of issues that used to be part of an ordinary life. Some salient cases include baldness, lower libido, shyness, bad temper, and difficulty getting pregnant.

On most occasions, overdiagnosis results from a combination of several reasons, with vast implications. A clear example is a condition known as attention deficit hyperactivity disorder, or ADHD, which was diagnosed in 2 million more American children and adolescents in 2011 than in 2003. The extent of the problem is so big that more than 20 percent of high-school-age boys in the US in 2011 were told they had ADHD. At the same time, almost 30 percent of people diagnosed as having asthma do not have it. In Australia, 18 percent of all cancers diagnosed in women (11,000 cases each year) and 24 percent of those in men (18,000 annually) are overdiagnosed, including 73 percent of people mislabeled as having thyroid cancer.

AVOIDING OVERTREATMENT

Asking "What is enough?" becomes vital when in the hands of medical professionals, especially when more aggressive measures that go beyond testing and diagnostics are being suggested. American physicians estimate that 21 percent of what they do to patients is unnecessary. This includes 1 of every 5 medications they prescribe and more than 1 in 10 procedures they perform. The main reasons relate closely to patients' behavior toward physicians. They may overtreat out of fear of being sued for malpractice (85 percent) or because of pressure or requests from patients to have procedures done (59 percent). Most physicians are also more likely to perform unnecessary procedures when they profit from them.

As absurd as it may sound, it is significantly safer to board a spacecraft, a nuclear submarine, or even a commercial airplane than it is to be admitted to a US hospital. There are around 98,000 unnecessary deaths in US hospitals annually as a result of errors. Even though this number is likely an underestimate, it is much higher than the number of deaths related to diabetes, influenza, or suicide. Surgeons can play a large role in reducing these rates, namely by avoiding operations that are not needed, not indicated, or not in the patient's best interest when weighed against other available options. This is something that has been widely known for decades within the medical world, where it has been acknowledged that the public would be shocked if it knew the number of unnecessary surgeries performed. Those for pain relief and weight loss are the most frequent, where 78 percent and 71 percent, respectively, of patients undergoing sham surgeries report improvements. Even spinal fusions, mainly for back pain, have been shown not to lead to improved long-term patient outcomes when compared with nonoperative treatments, including physical therapy and core strengthening exercises.

COPING WITH INFORMATION OVERLOAD

What is enough in terms of information? Can there be too much?

For most of the past 100,000 years, humans created, distributed, shared, and exchanged information at a pace that remained within the boundaries of our capacity to process and use it. In the 15th century, the situation started to change rapidly. With the introduction, development, and widespread use of the printing press, our ability to produce and distribute information accelerated and quickly outpaced our capacity to handle it.

The medical industrial complex is a perfect microcosm of this. Even in the early 1990s, before the explosion of digital technologies, research confirmed that busy physicians did not have enough time to read all the relevant information in their disciplines. The prime example was internal medicine, which had about 20 clinical journals at the time. To keep up, a dedicated doctor would have needed to read about 17 articles a day every day of the year. A decade later, the estimate for primary care practitioners was 14 times higher, and they would have needed more than 20 hours every day to read the relevant material.

With the hyperproduction and hyperdistribution of health-related content that digital technologies made possible, very soon the general public was also drowning in billions of pieces of information, available through an exploding number of devices and channels. Although this unprecedented amount of information can enable savvy people to become better informed around challenges of concern to them, thus increasing their adaptability, in most cases the effect has been detrimental.

The catastrophic abundance of health-related information from so many sources can heighten people's perception of risk, adding to their stress and anxiety. It is especially harmful when they are facing a life-threatening situation and realize that they are unable to discern between real and fake material.

Information overload can also increase the TSL to the point that people become sad, frustrated, or angry, ultimately stopping their search for information or even avoiding it altogether. In other cases, a high TSL is compounded by an overreliance on information shared through digital social networks, which can trigger negative emotions and loss of trust, and feed conspiracy theories and social unrest. This can in turn undermine the relationship between the public and health professionals, who can easily become targets of violent attacks.

MODERATING IMPROVEMENTS

Along with the harmful oversupply of health-related information, rapid technological development has given birth to innumerable artificial options to augment or replace bodily functions altogether. The question of what is enough is highly relevant in this space as well.

The introduction of mechanical, electronic, and biological innovations in modern medicine that are able to alter biology, shape appearance, and bolster mental or physical functioning has opened the door to new possibilities to adapt to life's challenges. This in turn has led down the slope to "enhancement technologies," which are interventions intended to improve human function or characteristics beyond what is necessary to sustain health or repair the body.

The highest expressions of human technological enhancement happen through a movement called transhumanism. Members of this faction seek to replace natural evolution with deliberate efforts to increase the level of human adaptability. Their pursuits are focused on tools that will be permanently integrated into the human body to boost human physical, emotional, cognitive, and behavioral functions as a means to improve human health and to extend human life spans.

So where is the limit in terms of changing bodies and enhancing minds? Some may say that the limit should be immortality itself. Others are emboldened by what has been called amortality, the belief that it is possible to forestall aging and to avoid or ignore decrepitude and death.

Not so fast, says another group of researchers. They offer evidence suggesting that even if we were able to eliminate things that usually kill us, our body's capacity to deal with challenges and adapt would fade with time. Even if we have the easiest life, this incremental decline seems to set the maximum life span for humans at between 120 and 150 years. If this is so, the only way to extend our lives indefinitely would be through means that transcend our original genetic programming, as well as our human bodies and mental faculties, purportedly with the use of synthetic biology and avatars or by blending ourselves with machines. At that point, we would find ourselves in the post-human era, where our current notions of self-reported health, personhood, or even the human species would be irrelevant.

This shows, perfectly, how sometimes when considering the question "What is enough?" it is not always up to you. It is nice to think that this is in your control. However, on many occasions that is not the case. You may have no say at all.

Who Decides?

According to longevity research, sometimes our biology decides how much is enough. In other instances, excesses must be handled by institutions. The medical systems of the members of the Organisation for Economic Co-operation and Development (OECD) concluded in 2017 that about one-third of total expenditures are wasted. In the US, the leader in catastrophic abundance, estimates in 2012 were as high as 50 percent.

What has been done to deal with this problem? Driven by the need to curb overtesting, overdiagnosis, and overtreatment, ambitious initiatives have been launched to offer clinicians and patients resources to assist them in making decisions in every clinical setting. One of these initiatives is Choosing Wisely, launched in 2012 in the US. It spread quickly to other countries and led to the identification of more than 1,000 opportunities to reduce costs and harms in its first decade.

In some ways, our biological opponents may be the ones deciding how much is enough. A major global concern is the overuse of antibiotics, which in half of all cases are inappropriately prescribed. On top of that, up to 90 percent of these prescriptions are inappropriately consumed by members of the public. There is also overuse of antibiotics in animals. Taken together, these situations have far-reaching severe consequences. The more antibiotics are used, the more bacteria become resistant to them. As this occurs, the list of infections that used to be easily cured but now are hard or impossible to treat is growing at an alarming rate.

What are the main implications of this? Humans are at risk of losing the evolutionary competition with disease-producing bacteria. Because of our shortsightedness, our adversaries are being allowed to adapt to our most effective tools designed to control them. As many as 7 percent of deaths worldwide are associated with bacterial resistance. Young children in hospitals, especially those under 5 years of age, are most at risk: One in five of their deaths are linked to it. This situation is compounded by the detrimental lack of new antibiotics, resulting from both the absence of financial incentives for pharmaceutical companies to develop novel solutions and the neglectful actions of most governments around the world, which are unwilling to fill the gap. This vulnerability persists even in the face of repeated global resolutions acknowledging the risks posed by the superbugs that are threatening the survival of the species. These bacteria are essentially dictating how much medicine is enough, with disastrous consequences if we go over or under the level they set.

Reaching "Enoughness"

What can you do to protect yourself from the devastating consequences of too much medicine and make your way toward enough? One of the most powerful and yet difficult things that anyone can do to face these challenges is to go to the root of the problem and address the issue of insatiability at the individual level.

Insatiability is also seen as something that can be managed, to a certain extent, through self-transformation within the family setting. This might be the only feasible option to reach the sweet spot needed to trigger "enoughness" on a large scale.

The chances of success will likely increase if you follow a strategy that involves figuring out what to believe or ignore and noticing how enoughness feels.

WHAT TO BELIEVE

The first hurdle to overcome is the belief that more is more. Given the consistently dismal figures related to too much medicine, it would be sensible to strive for less testing and less treatment to reach the point of enough of both.

How much is enough in this sense? The best approach to answer this question for yourself is to access materials from the growing number of patient-led organizations that are producing evidence-based materials in easy-to-understand language. Such materials will likely dispel a lot of your beliefs—for instance, that you need an MRI if you just hurt your lower back; or that antibiotics work against a cold, even though most colds are produced by viruses rather than bacteria.

In questioning what to believe, it is vital to learn how to spot fake news—misinformation that is deliberately created and spread via any kind of media. Within the medical sphere, fake news is often produced and distributed with the intention of damaging an organization, group, or person, or to profit from people's fears and gullibility. Its creators often use exaggerated, sensationalist headlines and content that is slanted or deceptive, and sometimes outright false. This content is usually motivated by the financial interests of those who are trying to sell you more of something you value: more beauty, more physical strength, more sexual vitality, more mental capacity, more peace of mind. Although it is practically impossible to distinguish the best fake pieces from trustworthy information, most can be detected by asking yourself a couple of questions: Is the information reinforcing my urges? Will those who produced it profit from my compliance?

Even when you consider the source to be reputable, it can be helpful to ask the following questions before making any serious decisions:

- When was this information published?
- Is it clear which information sources were used (other than the author or producer)?
- Does the piece contain information about risks?
- Does it include or mention alternatives?

EXPERIENCING ENOUGH

Reaching the sweet spot of enough requires recognizing that you do not have a fixed list of desires and that some of those you do have can be problematic. Sometimes they are simply dissatisfying placeholders for things that are unattainable. In the medical space, immortality of the physical body appears to be impossible, and so insatiability runs rampant in the form of futile surgeries, pills, creams, and procedures.

With this understanding and knowing that more tends to be less beneficial to your adaptability than in ancient times, it is crucial to have self-compassion and accept that experiencing enoughness requires looking inward.

Answering the question "What is enough?" is similar to that of self-reported health in that it aggregates and distills a wide range of complex data points into a graspable and actionable conclusion. The main source of information may actually be inside of you, signals that are known colloquially as your "gut feelings." These are interoceptive sensations generated by many tissues in your body that are capable of influencing your behaviors and decisions, including your gut, but also your heart, lungs, and skin. Although these signals are mostly unconscious and on the fringes of your awareness, they have been shown to be valuable in making risky decisions, such as those made by gamblers, financial traders, and surgeons. In other words, if something inside of you gives you the sense that you are doing too much or have too much, pay attention. Conversely, if you have a feeling of enoughness, take notice and try to maintain it. This is your internal compass, directing you toward the right balance. It is almost like the sense of magnetic north that birds and a long list of other animals have, which they rely on to navigate the skies, the seas, and the land.

Your answers to this question about enough are key to enhancing your efforts to adapt and thrive. They can lead to new and healthier habits, while making the limits of what is right for you clearer. This extra level of awareness can also make it easier for you to recognize that the sense of enough is like a boundary, and if you cross it, you may hurt yourself or others.

On occasion, your evaluation of what is enough could justify a visit to a medical facility or the need to come into contact with medical professionals. In these situations, your sense of enoughness will be critical as a powerful navigational tool to find your way in such an essential and yet dangerous space. You will also need to have a deeper understanding of how the system works so that you can evade its plentiful fatal traps and enjoy optimal results.

CHAPTER 11

SURVIVING THE MEDICAL INDUSTRIAL COMPLEX

t is often said, tongue in cheek, that for the medical system, "health is a state of incomplete diagnosis." The chances of being diagnosed with one or more diseases increase with every visit to a doctor. In the US alone, people make a total of 860 million trips to see a physician annually, with 86 percent of adults and 96 percent of children having at least one appointment.

A survey of 2,000 people in the UK estimated that on average, a person will experience, over a lifetime of 81 years, 729 cuts and bumps, 810 headaches, 405 bouts of heartburn or indigestion, 405 colds and sore throats, 324 episodes of back pain, 243 pulled or strained muscles, 162 episodes of neck pain, and 81 toothaches, as well as 4 hospital admissions, 2 surgeries, and 1 broken bone.

In sum, there are plenty of opportunities for you to be regarded as a "patient" at any stage of your life. The question is, how can you play the best possible role and get superior results from your encounters with the medical industrial complex?

Becoming a Good Patient

In medicine, the notion of a "good patient" has traditionally been judged by healthcare providers. The limited literature on this subject indicates that this designation is usually given to someone who is considered "interesting" because their clinical characteristics challenge the physician's skills. In addition, a "traditional good patient" is someone who acknowledges the physician's expertise and complies passively with the doctor's orders and recommendations as the main path to getting well enough to return to their usual social roles. This reflects the fact that at least until the last quarter of the 20th century, patients were viewed as helpless, vulnerable, irrational, and docile. They were considered as being dependent on a benevolent medical establishment, with minimal expected involvement in their own care. This was mainly because they were seen as not competent enough to help themselves, or even to know what needed to be done or how to do it.

This role has evolved. More modern perspectives value an increasingly active role by patients, especially when they talk with healthcare professionals about their illnesses, provided that they are neither "belligerent nor demanding." Clinicians also regard as "good" those patients who ask "appropriate" and "respectful" questions that reflect their understanding of biomedical issues, and who show "gratitude" and "respect."

Those who do not conform to these roles are "bad patients," who might even be fired by their physicians. The main reasons for this happening, at least in the US, are exhibiting "difficult behaviors associated with mental illness," failing to pay medical bills, missing "too many" appointments, failing to follow recommended care, and continuing "to misbehave."

How to evaluate whether a patient is good or bad has historically been determined by healthcare professionals withaout taking into consideration the views, wants, or needs of their patients. But what happens when a physician becomes a patient?

We decided to pursue this question by asking a couple of physicians to describe what they experienced when they had to interact with the healthcare system as patients. This turned out to be a very powerful exercise, because their conclusions about what is involved in being a good patient changed radically when they switched roles.

This exploration led to the identification of five key insights about how it is possible for patients to get better results from the healthcare system. They have since been regarded as essential for "the good patient of the future." They are all supported by strong scientific evidence, and in most cases, it is possible to put them into action without increasing costs, requiring more time, or needing fancy technologies. It only takes an assertive patient and a confident healthcare provider who is willing to listen.

1. ENSURE THAT YOUR MAIN QUESTIONS ARE ANSWERED

Many patients leave the doctor's office, clinic, or virtual consultation or enter the operating room with unanswered questions, mostly because of what has been labeled "white-coat silence." This is a phenomenon produced by the anxiety, and strong sense of intimidation, vulnerability, and inadequacy, generated by the unfamiliar surroundings, the long waits, the strange faces, and the impotence experienced by patients in most healthcare settings, especially when dealing with a high-stakes situation or a potentially life-threatening condition. It is made worse by the limited time patients usually have available to interact with physicians, which is around 5 minutes per encounter in half of the world—averaging from 48 seconds in Bangladesh to 22.5 minutes in Sweden. In half of all encounters, it takes just 11 seconds for patients to be interrupted by their doctors.

Surprisingly, when you are given the opportunity to ask questions in your own way, actual consultation time does not increase, but you leave feeling more satisfied and feeling that you have spent more time with the doctor.

Making a list of important questions before a consultation will help ensure that you won't forget anything important. Asking the questions (and getting answers) can make you feel less anxious and more satisfied. You are also more likely to get better. The effects seem to be greater when you make a list yourself, without coaching or prompting, than when you are given an existing menu of questions from which to choose.

2. DECIDE HOW MUCH YOU WILL PARTICIPATE IN DECISIONS ABOUT YOUR MEDICAL CARE

You have the right and the responsibility to decide for yourself how active a role you want to play in decisions about your healthcare. Your role may change, if necessary, at different points during your interactions with the medical industrial complex.

You may want that role to be small ("The doctor knows best; I'd like her to decide for me"), or you may wish for almost complete autonomy ("Give me the facts, and I'll decide for myself"). You may also prefer to be given the relevant information and make particular decisions jointly with your healthcare provider. Alternatively, you might choose an approach we designed called "collaborative decision making," which would enable you, your loved ones, and any professional involved in your care to engage in a joint process aimed at achieving positive health, according to your own preferences, values, and circumstances.

There is a significant association between positive health and active involvement in the decision-making process. Nevertheless, although it should be up to you to decide, the medical industrial complex gives patients only about a one in three chance to participate in decisions about their care in the ways they prefer.

Commonly, you will have a more reduced role in the decision-making process than you might wish. To overcome this risk, you must state your preference to the professionals involved in your care, or in the care of a loved one, whenever a big decision is about to be made, so that you can all work toward achieving a positive level of self-reported health together.

3. ENSURE THAT YOU KNOW WHAT IS GOING ON BETWEEN EPISODES OF CARE

Whenever you enter the healthcare system with declining levels of health, you will likely be exposed to critical information about your diagnosis, treatment options, and prognosis, and given instructions that you might easily forget, misinterpret, or not comprehend, with serious consequences.

The more information you receive, the more you will likely forget. In fact, 40 to 80 percent of the medical information patients receive is forgotten immediately, and almost half of what is remembered is recalled incorrectly.

Scientific evidence also suggests that people with low levels of health literacy—namely, insufficient skills to access, understand, and use information in ways that promote and maintain good health—are admitted to the hospital and end up in the emergency room more often, report greater levels of negative health, and experience higher premature mortality rates from all causes. It has been shown that each percentage increase in low health literacy within a community is associated with a 2 percent increase in poor self-reported health.

Stress and anxiety also impair the capacity of a person to recall relevant information. Most patients with a life-threatening diagnosis tend to struggle to retrieve information about their treatment. This is likely most pronounced among older cancer patients, who have been shown to remember only 20 percent of the instructions for when to call their healthcare provider, 23 percent of the recommendations for how to deal with side effects, and 27 percent of the suggestions for how to reduce the impact of chemotherapy on their daily lives.

Getting information verbally is a poor way for patients to ensure that they will understand and accurately remember vital information, especially when they are alone. It has been shown, consistently, that the level of understanding of what is happening and what should be done and why increases significantly, for both patients and their companions, when healthcare professionals provide written summaries or recordings of their encounters.

Involving trusted people as companions is also paramount, especially in stressful encounters with the healthcare system, as they can facilitate asking questions, take notes, and help recall information, particularly when making important decisions about treatment options.

4. GET A SINGLE POINT OF CONTACT WITH THE HEALTHCARE SYSTEM

Successfully navigating the healthcare system, especially when feeling anxious because of one or more health-related challenges, demands much more than understanding the information that is given. In most cases, you receive services from multiple providers working across several locations, who often use incompatible digital platforms to manage clinical or administrative data, or who simply have disparate ways of running their practices. Having to navigate such a fragmented landscape—alone or even with a committed companion who is unfamiliar with the healthcare system—can add to your toxic stress load, increasing the likelihood that you will experience negative health levels, suboptimal outcomes, and avoidable complications, while wasting valuable resources.

Although the recognition of the negative consequences of fragmented, poorly integrated healthcare systems has driven a push in most countries to increase the level of integration of service providers, evidence suggests that it is more important to coordinate care around your needs than to integrate all the services at your disposal. For that reason, you are better off with providers who make an effort to "hide the wiring" so that you can experience seamless care, regardless of what happens behind the scenes. When this is done well, the system itself benefits too. When providers and services are coordinated to yield a smooth patient experience, it is possible to see a 27 percent drop in the number of visits to the emergency room, 13 percent fewer hospital admissions, and a 17 percent reduction in costs.

A very practical and effective way to improve service coordination, and above all patient satisfaction, is to have a single point of contact with the medical industrial complex. This is usually achieved through the engagement of a person who is designated as a "care coordinator," "case manager," or "navigator." Such a person does not need to have a clinical background or specialized training, but good interpersonal skills and knowledge of the inner workings of the patient's healthcare service ecosystem are important, as is the authority to get things done by all the relevant system players. In situations where this role does not exist formally, a caring nurse or social worker can usually fill the gap.

5. REQUEST A SECOND OPINION

Second opinions are usually considered by patients who are facing a life-threatening disease, when the original doctor is unable to provide a diagnosis for a potentially serious illness or recommends a major procedure, or when all treatments that have been offered have failed to produce the desired effects. Requesting a second opinion can be difficult, however, as the patient may feel embarrassed or afraid that it will weaken their relationship with their doctor or create ill feelings. To overcome this hurdle, several countries, starting with Germany in 2015, have legislated the right to a second opinion at no cost to the patient. Research supports this move.

When important clinical decisions are reassessed by cancer specialists, the diagnosis, treatment recommendations, or prognosis may change in up to 69 percent of cases, with almost 60 percent of all discrepancies categorized as major. In addition, up to 95 percent of patients report a high satisfaction level with second opinions, feeling that receiving another opinion helps them gain greater understanding of their treatment options (93 percent), their illness (88 percent), and the risks of the treatment (82 percent). A similar picture emerges from the data in relation to other major decisions. Only one-third of recommendations for orthopedic surgery are confirmed when a case is reviewed by a second specialist, who is likely to suggest noninvasive, cheaper, or less risky interventions instead.

The picture is even more dramatic when deciding whether it

is necessary to undergo an angiography—a type of X-ray procedure used to check the blood vessels that feed the heart. A careful assessment of second opinions led to the conclusion that
50 percent of these tests performed in the US are unnecessary, or
at least could be postponed.

Avoiding Preventable Harm

The medical industrial complex is full of additional possibilities
to cause harm, even when you are armed with these five insights.
Every decision, no matter what is involved, has risks. The main
issue, however, is whether such harm is preventable, namely
whether there is a clear cause for it and whether you, or anyone
else, can do anything about it.

An extensive analysis of 70 studies mostly conducted in the
US and Europe concluded that around 12 percent of patients
experience harm when in contact with the medical industrial
complex. In other words, one of every eight patients will suffer
"unanticipated, unforeseen accidents (e.g., patient injuries, care
complications, or death) which are a direct result of the care dis-
pensed rather than the patient's underlying disease." Of these,
half are preventable (6 percent, or 1 in 18 patients).

Most of the preventable harm is caused by drugs (25 percent), followed by surgery (23 percent) and infections and diagnostic tests (16 percent each). Harm is most often experienced
by children and older adults and tends to occur more frequently
in the most sophisticated medical facilities, especially in the in-
tensive care units of advanced hospitals. In 9 to 15 percent
of cases, the patient is left with a persistent disability or dies.
This means that 1 of every 100 to 200 patients is seriously

harmed by the healthcare system or dies from causes that could be avoided.

What is at the root of so much preventable harm? It can be linked directly to factors associated with a lack—manifested as ignorance, inexperience, incompetence, negligence, and corruption. There is little that patients can do about these factors in most cases. Nevertheless, they can reduce the risk associated with getting the wrong medication while in the hospital by double-checking the label themselves and confirming the right dose on the spot. It might also be beneficial for patients to ask healthcare workers whether they have washed their hands. Even though that might sound like a minor point and it might be an embarrassing question to ask, handwashing can have an important effect on the reduction of preventable infections and deaths. Despite being a proven, simple, highly effective, and fully understood practice, less than half of healthcare professionals wash their hands before coming in contact with patients.

Similarly, patients can reduce the risk of being operated on in the wrong place by marking the precise spot for the procedure or reminding the surgeon of the type of surgery that is supposed to be performed before being anesthetized. Is this actually necessary? Yes. Twenty-one percent of hand surgeons have made this mistake, with 80 percent of the cases involving surgery on the wrong finger. Twenty-five percent of neurosurgeons report having started operations by cutting on the wrong side of the head, and 35 percent at the wrong level of the back.

Beyond minimizing the latent risk of preventable harm, which is always there, how can you experience the highest possible levels of positive health while interacting with the medical industrial complex?

Making Possible What Is Possible

Matching what you need with what medicine can be expected to deliver can play a big role in your achieving a high level of positive health.

CURING THE CURABLE

The power to get rid of diseases is the main selling point of the medical industrial complex, and possibly the prime justification for the vast resources it consumes every year. However, one of the best-kept secrets is that this is possible only within a narrow menu of options. The clearest example, and the dominant one, is the use of antimicrobials for infections. Antimicrobials are chemical compounds that can kill microorganisms such as bacteria, fungi, viruses, and parasites. When they are used effectively, they produce the clearest evidence of a "cure," as patients no longer have a particular germ.

Medicine can also claim the power to cure diseases through surgery, particularly when it is possible to remove all the tissue in the body that is affected by a disease. This is typically applicable to cancerous lesions that are localized within a very specific part of the body—say, the skin or the breast. Surgery can also cure other diseases by replacing the affected body parts using transplants or prostheses; by reconstructing body parts that are damaged, as with hernias; or by removing objects that are causing distressing symptoms, such as stones in the kidneys or gallbladder.

Besides antimicrobials and surgery, medicine can claim to be the main party responsible for cures in emergency situations that involve bodily injuries, such as those caused by physical trauma (e.g., a bone fracture) or poisonous substances. It can also "fix" a growing number of problems by correcting genetic defects or boosting the body's defenses (e.g., using immunotherapy).

Beyond these issues, the case for medicine to be the sole party or the main player responsible for curing ailments is weak. Other sectors, fields, and disciplines can claim similar or even greater power to improve levels of self-reported health. This is the case with diseases that can be corrected with supplements, such as anemia caused by vitamin deficiencies; mental disorders that can be corrected through psychotherapy, with or without professional involvement; and socially undesirable conditions such as baldness, which can be remedied with hair implants.

The apparently large number of health challenges that are "fixable" pales in comparison with the number that are not. In this context, medicine finds itself on even shakier ground to justify its preeminent role as a contributor to human health.

MANAGING THE MANAGEABLE

An even better-kept secret is that most of the funding that the medical industrial complex receives is devoted not to curing diseases, but to dealing with challenges that are unfixable. These tend to be labeled as "non-communicable diseases" or "chronic diseases" and include every pathological condition that is not an infection, that does not go away for years, and that cannot be cured (yet) by medical means.

These diseases affect 45 percent of American adults and are responsible for 9 out of 10 deaths every year in the US, rates that are higher than the global average. The most common chronic diseases are dental cavities and gum inflammation, cancer, diabetes, stroke, heart disease, respiratory disease, and arthritis, which collectively account for nearly 75 percent of all of the healthcare spending in the country and consume 83 percent and 96 percent of the budgets of Medicaid and Medicare in the US, respectively. Across the world, they are also the leading causes of human mortality, responsible for 60 percent of all deaths annually. This rate keeps increasing as the dietary habits, psychological stress, and sedentary behaviors that come with "Western" ways of life are adopted by societies throughout the globe, and as their deadly competitor, infections, becomes less lethal.

Chronic diseases are also the leading cause of long-term disability for humans, with about a quarter of patients reporting severe disease and a third reporting negative health at any given time. Most people (80 percent) with chronic conditions rarely have only one, with 48 percent of those 65 years of age or older living with three or more.

Half of the patients with three or more chronic conditions report negative health. This creates a major challenge for the healthcare system, which in most places organizes its services into groups devoted to specific organs (e.g., the heart) or diseases (e.g., cancer), with poor communication among them.

Given that chronic conditions are incurable, all that medicine can offer are diagnostic tests and medications. Rarely are patients given options drawn from the 90 percent of the choices found outside the medical industrial complex. Thus, many people (between 40 and 60 percent) in high-income countries, including the US, take five or more prescription drugs on a daily basis. All of these "solutions" may be for nothing: In 40 percent of cases, such drugs are unnecessary. Piling on, these futile prescriptions could actually be increasing the risk of preventable harm from adverse effects, regardless of the drugs involved. In addition, often as a means to control the side effects of prescribed drugs, even more medication is added, without any changes to the older ones or any formal assessment of whether they are producing their intended results or doing more harm than good.

Considering this, what can be done to manage this situation? It is crucial for patients to enlist a healthcare provider, either a physician or a nurse, in a process known as deprescribing, which seeks to reduce and stop, gradually and systematically, the number of inappropriate medications they take. A review of multiple studies on deprescription showed that it can reduce premature deaths by up to 70 percent. The researchers did not find a single case of increased mortality resulting from reducing the number of drugs patients take.

How does deprescribing work? The first step is to separate the drugs according to whether they intend to "control the controllable" (e.g., risk factors, such as high blood pressure, cholesterol, and sugar levels, or the progression of the disease itself) or to "relieve the relievable" (e.g., symptoms such as pain, shortness of breath, and fatigue). Then, based on the patient's preferences and priorities, a joint decision is made as to which drugs to keep and which to discontinue, ideally complemented by non-pharmacological alternatives (e.g., increases in physical activity and dietary changes).

ACCEPTING THE INEVITABLE

The medicalization of life, which focuses either on curing diseases or on offering medical responses to psychological and social challenges, has tried to brush aside or ignore what might be the most important challenge of all: how to be healthy until the very end of life.

We tried to gain insights about this by reviewing all the research on what it would take to die well, from the perspective of the healthcare system. We found 11 themes that have been described consistently over decades in different regions of the world. When their time comes, people would like to (1) die at their preferred place (most often their own home), (2) be free from pain and other physical symptoms, (3) get relief from emotional distress and other forms of psychological suffering, (4) receive emotional support from their loved ones, (5) make autonomous decisions about any treatment they might receive, (6) circumvent futile life-prolonging interventions, (7) avoid being a burden to others, (8) have the right to assisted suicide or euthanasia, (9) be capable of engaging in effective communication with healthcare professionals, (10) take part in rituals of value to them, and (11) be aware of the deep significance of what is happening. All of these were endorsed by more than 3,000 physicians and other healthcare professionals whom we asked what conditions they would like to find at the end of their lives to consider their own deaths to be good.

What is noteworthy about these findings is that hardly any of these conditions require medical expertise or sophisticated infrastructure. What they demand instead is a willingness to re-imagine the role of medicine and to mobilize all the resources available, within and beyond the healthcare system, especially those that might otherwise be regarded as unrelated to health, so that everyone can have the greatest chance to experience what truly matters: a long and healthy life until the last breath.

Achieving this goal requires the skills needed to deal with what is yet to happen. And guess what? You already have those skills.

CHAPTER 12

YOU ARE A FORMIDABLE MARVEL

C an you say, with absolute certainty, whether you will be healthy at 3:00 P.M. next Sunday?

Whether it is Monday, Tuesday, or any other day of the week, it does not matter if you do not know. It is irrelevant. Whatever happens, you will be able to handle it. You are equipped to face any situation. Why? Because you have a superpower and a defense system to take on both known and unknown challenges. This superpower is your adaptability, and the defense system is everything that makes you adaptable. Together they are like a divine gift protecting you from practically anything and everything that could harm you or make you not healthy. They have been refined over the billions of years since life began on earth, developing through practically infinite interactions and trial and error. You are the end result of all of that. You are a dynamic, flexible, formidable marvel.

Throughout this book, we have explored the various expressions of this indivisible whole. Everything mentioned is interconnected. The idea of individual pieces, which follow a particular sequence, is an illusion. There is no such thing as "inside" or "outside" (in the same way that trees are part of your respiratory system), with every aspect vital to the totality (rather than being optional).

Your adapt-ability makes whatever comes next to challenge you almost irrelevant. After all, it is the way in which you adjust in response to novel, changing, unknown, unexpected, or uncertain circumstances, so as to become better suited to thrive under new conditions. It allows you to react to change itself, rather than to specific threats.

You are equipped culturally, socially, psychologically, and physically to do most of your adapting without noticing. Most of your challenges require low-energy responses and are fielded by unnoticeable mechanisms—homeostasis, allostasis, interoception, exteroception, and proprioception. Even your obliviousness to most of what is going on showcases the elegant efficiency of your defense system. Whenever challenges do appear on your radar, such elegance allows you to respond in the most energy-efficient way, ranging from doing nothing to dissolving or removing the challenge altogether. When the responses that require lower levels of energy become ineffective, you can boost your capacity to react by parsing out the elements of a challenge into categories (physical, psychological, or social). This can help you address any situation with or without aid from others.

Remember, you feel more than you know. It is astounding that by just taking 10 seconds to answer a question about how healthy you feel, you can get a grasp of your prospects for living or losing 20 years of life. Rating your own health as negative can triple your risk of dying earlier than your peers who rate their health as positive. Therefore, feeling that your health is "poor" or "fair" is an emergency requiring immediate attention. In this case, you will likely require professional support to avoid fatal consequences.

The predictive power of self-rating your health is high because you have an inner sense of what is happening inside your body and in the world around it. Self-rating is like a very sensitive barometer, capable of aggregating multiple complex inputs almost instantaneously. It becomes invaluable to guide your decisions about what to do next. You can check your health frequently by answering the following three questions, which will take less than one minute in most situations:

- In general, how would you rate your health: excellent, very good, good, fair, or poor?
- Why do you consider your health to be at that level?
- What do you need to maintain or improve your level of health?

Your answers can also reflect the state of trillions of microbes that share their lives with you. Instead of being a separate organism, you are the host of a large, rich, intimately entangled ecosystem made up of a small fraction of human cells, which are vastly outnumbered by cells and genetic material from different kingdoms, called your microbiome. These are key members of your defense system and your adaptability, leading the responses to potentially harmful invaders. They are part of your armed forces, participating in attacks against other microorganisms that can cause infections. They can also create physical and chemical barriers to protect you from diseases. Although they are most numerous in the gut, they are also present throughout your body. Thus, your human cells and your microbiome form a much greater whole that cannot be separated. You are much more than you might have thought. Considering yourself as a separate individual is an oversimplification; you are a holobiont.

When you feel that you need to boost these tiny allies, you

can add to and nourish them with "functional foods" and in some cases a fecal transplant. After all, they contribute significantly to how you rate your health, which ultimately says a lot about how well and for how long you will live.

They also influence the "gut feelings" that help you answer another essential question: What is enough? (This is an invaluable reflection when you are navigating the medical industrial complex, especially to protect yourself from too much medicine.) Similar to what happens when you assess your own levels of health, this question aggregates and distills a wide range of complex interoceptive sensations generated by many tissues in your body that can influence your behaviors and decisions. Although these signals are mostly unconscious and at the fringes of your awareness, they have been shown to be valuable in making risky decisions, such as those made by gamblers, financial traders, and surgeons.

Your feeling of enoughness is your internal compass, directing you toward the right balance. It is almost like the sense of magnetic north that a long list of animals have, which they rely on to navigate the skies, the seas, and the land. In other words, if something inside of you gives you the sense that you are doing too much or have too much, pay attention. The extra degrees of awareness that you will gain by checking your levels of health and enoughness could be invaluable as you attempt to tame the fear of disease, curb overtesting, contain overdiagnosis, avoid overtreatment, cope with information overload, and make decisions about the myriad temptations you will experience to improve your body and mind.

On any occasion, based on your self-evaluations of health and enoughness, you may notice that further action is needed. In these moments, it could be useful to remember that your defense system also includes other people, as well as your links with them and how they connect with one another. Just as is the case with the interactions between your human and microbial cells, your relationships with other people in your network generate novel patterns, properties, and behaviors that make the whole more than the sum of its parts.

The people around you, those whom you consider your friends, and the networks in which they are embedded can protect you when you are facing a challenge. Friendship is so powerful that it has been regarded as "the single most important factor influencing our health, well-being, and happiness." For this power to manifest fully, it is crucial that you carefully choose whom you call "friend." In ideal circumstances, these are the people you like, respect, appreciate, and trust. Typically, you will spend 60 percent of your social time with your 15 "best friends." Ideally, your closest group will have ties that are so special that you could regard one another as members of a family by choice. With this "created" or "chosen" family at the core of your personal social network, you will all have an adaptive advantage in times of hardship by providing one another with physical, emotional, and practical social support whenever and wherever you need it.

A family by choice can be the main way to combat loneliness, which has become an existential threat for humans. Another option is joining a proactive social network, allowing you to meet new people. Together you can build bonds while championing a cause or even diving deep into a hobby.

You also have the capacity to supercharge the adaptive potential of your personal social networks through digital tools, which can allow you to support and be supported by practically anyone else around the world. This level of access to the whole human network will take your capacity to adapt to almost any existing or new challenge to new heights.

It is also crucial to recognize that networks can be vehicles of social contagion, allowing the spread of ideas, attitudes, or behaviors from one person to another. These can be adaptive or maladaptive and can affect you at a distance, even through people you do not know, such as the friends of your friends' friends.

No matter what you go through, most encounters with challenges leave behind scars, tensions, and burdens that pile up, which we call the toxic stress load. When your TSL becomes overwhelming, your response to ongoing or new challenges can become maladaptive, causing more harm than the challenges themselves. A high TSL triggers changes so profound that they are equivalent to accelerated aging. An excessive TSL is also associated with risky behaviors, such as poor eating habits, physical inactivity, tobacco smoking, excessive alcohol consumption, abuse of other drugs, and inadequate sleep patterns. These behaviors feed a lethal cycle, contributing to higher rates of cancer, stroke, depression, suicidal ideation, post-traumatic stress disorder, seizures, obesity, diabetes, and asthma. The TSL is what can ultimately kill you early. It is one of the biggest challenges for those pushing the limits of longevity.

Nobody can go through life completely free of a TSL. Yours began to build up when you were inside your mother's womb, and possibly even before your parents were born, and will stop affecting you only when you die. Luck has a lot to do with how high your TSL is and how quickly it accumulates, and how well you will handle it during your life. You will also be profoundly affected by the place where you were born and the labels that were assigned to you at birth. Even so, regardless of how fortunate or unfortunate you have been, there is a lot that you can do to influence your TSL. Studies of extraordinarily long-lived people provide many hopeful lessons. They validate separate research on the importance that physical activity, eating habits, smoking, and alcohol use can have on your health and longevity. They also confirm the power of personal social networks to prevent loneliness and to nurture close family relationships and strong friendships.

The insights from those who are pushing the limits of human longevity and health also echo the findings of research on the benefits of the spaces where your life unfolds. Fortunately, there is a rich and wide variety of settings that we have grouped by color to make it easier for you to make the most of them. In particular, Green Spaces—anywhere you are exposed to vegetation—can help you reduce your TSL by lowering your stress level, lifting your mood, and improving your sleep quality. Some of these effects can be transferred into your bedroom or office by adding something as apparently simple as a plant, which can also purify the air and control mold. In optimal circumstances, exposure to plants has been shown to reduce the odds of premature death by one-third.

You will also find, by contrast, that Red Spaces are frequent sources of challenges, especially because they are the settings where many of your interactions with the medical industrial complex will occur. Some of these challenges emanate from the design of the spaces themselves, as most institutions tend to be built as featureless production lines for diagnosing, curing, and treating diseases. This is why almost all of the clinics or hospitals you will visit are likely to increase your levels of anxiety and stress, unless you are fortunate enough to find one of the few that are truly attempting to become healing places.

The majority of the challenges you will face in Red Spaces relate to the services provided by medical facilities. One of the most important ones is to resist the urge to visit a doctor in the first place. Given that 90 percent of what you need to experience positive health is nonmedical, you should use the medical industrial complex for what it does best: deal with acute and life-threatening problems, such as heart attacks and strokes, major injuries from accidents, infections, and severe pain. It can also be the most appropriate setting to manage a condition that needs a prescription or undergo an intervention that only a doctor can perform.

You should also consider using the medical industrial complex whenever you rate your health as negative, when you feel "off," or when your levels of positive health begin decreasing rapidly. In any of those cases, five key insights can increase your chances of getting the best possible results from the medical system and protect you or your loved ones from avoidable harm:

1. Ensure that your main questions are answered.
2. Decide how much you will participate in decisions about your medical care.
3. Ensure that you know what is going on between episodes of care.
4. Get a single point of contact with the healthcare system.
5. Request a second opinion.

These guiding principles can also help you avoid too much medicine. They can support you in ensuring that whatever is done by the medical system, to you or to your loved ones, is motivated by the explicit intention of curing the curable, managing the manageable, or accepting the inevitable.

Your risk of avoidable harm, however, extends beyond the medical industrial complex. Unfortunately, in many instances it is driven by your own Self-Destructive Force. This is your propensity to go against your better judgment and make decisions that you know will have negative consequences.

Trying to fight this force alone is usually futile. This is why creating a personal board of directors and relying on your personal network will give you the highest chances of success.

Your efforts to overcome your Self-Destructive Force, or any other factor contributing to your TSL, can be enhanced substantially by another tool in the arsenal of your defensive system: your capacity to build a healthy reality for yourself. Even something as simple as doing jumping jacks when you feel anxious can be very effective. The increased cardiac activity this produces can give your mind an opportunity to interpret a rapid heart rate as a harmless response to exercise, instead of relating it to something potentially catastrophic. Along similar lines, you can use digital tools designed to divert your attention away from negative thoughts and toward positive alternatives, or to make it easier for you to reject threatening thought patterns and replace them with positive interpretations of what is going on.

You, with all your abilities and tools, are truly amazing. It is exhilarating to see that you represent how human evolution has kept pushing the limits of what is possible and how you continue to find ways to thrive.

To go all the way and level up, there is one more aspect of your superpower of adaptability that can take you further. Just as you are able to deal with present challenges, you can overcome those that are yet to come even if you do not know what they are. Rather than freezing from your fear of uncertainty or feeling unsettled by the future, you can turn the unknown into something that will make you stronger and more able to be healthy, no matter what.

Come What May

You are always face-to-face with the unknowable. The only thing you know you can expect is change. How can you adapt to what is yet to happen so that you can feel healthy no matter what? How can you gain an advantage now over what may come next, regardless of what it might be?

One option was discovered by philosophers in ancient Greece more than 2,000 years ago. It is summed up by the expression "It's not what happens to you but how you react to it that matters." In other words, rather than trying to predict what is going to happen next, which is impossible, you can focus instead on responding in a way that will not add to your TSL. The original advocates of this approach chose a response that allowed them to be free from distress or worry, one that can be helpful for you to have as part of your adaptability arsenal. It is known as ataraxia, the feeling of deep tranquility or equanimity, with which you can react to whatever challenges you face in life.

A way to achieve ataraxia is by recognizing the initial effects that a challenge will have: On the one hand, you will perceive it as something that is happening to you. On the other hand, you will be compelled to label what is happening as bad and feel that change needs to occur. To free yourself from the distress that this produces, you will need to suspend your judgment about the "badness" of the perception, thus disabling its distressing potential.

Along the same lines is an approach to dealing with the unknown called *amor fati*, literally "love of fate." Rather than resigning yourself to an unchangeable future, this perspective involves having a positive outlook toward what is yet to happen. To achieve this, you must be prepared to welcome—with gratitude, loving kindness, and even cheerfulness—whatever the future might have in store for you. By doing so, instead of feeling trapped without any opportunity to change anything, you can experience freedom and tranquility in your commitment to love what is to come, regardless of what it is.

A complementary approach focuses on feeling comfortable that there are various ways to neutralize a challenge.

The first option for dealing with a challenge is to try to solve the underlying problem. This means that it is possible to find the causes of the challenge and eliminate them completely. As a result, the problem ends. In medicine, if you have an infection caused by bacteria, you take an antibiotic that can kill them—in the right dose and for a long enough time—and you are cured. The episode is over, but the problem can return.

The second option, when it is impossible to solve the underlying problem, is to try to manage its effects. This is done by tackling the symptoms that are causing you distress and adding to your TSL, and ideally any factor that can make the situation worse. This is what happens when a person has diabetes and is given insulin. The underlying problem continues, but it becomes tolerable or less harmful, at least for a while.

The third option, which many people do not consider, is a part of your superpower of adaptability. It allows you to make challenges vanish altogether. How can this be? You can dissolve a challenge by redesigning the context that makes it feel like a problem or by looking at the situation from a completely different angle, one in which the challenge ceases to exist as a problem. This is what happened with the reconceptualization of health. When health was reframed as the ability to adapt, the problems created by the original WHO definition of health essentially disappeared.

When it comes to adapting to future challenges, how can

you dissolve what seems to be the main problem: the uncertainty that is produced by their unknowability? The answer is what we call forecrafting, or the ability to make desirable imagined possibilities happen. When you forecraft, you are "presentifying" desirable possibilities. That is, you are aligning the future with what will eventually become the present. You do this, at least on a small scale and in the short term, as part of your daily life. This is what happens when you set an alarm clock and then wake up at the right time, or when you buy ingredients for a meal and then prepare something delicious. These examples are relatively simple and mostly depend on you, or things within your control.

To forecraft as a means of dissolving bigger challenges and at scale, you will need to unlearn many of the things you thought were expected or acceptable, and replace them with fresh insights and perspectives. In fact, your willingness and capacity to unlearn has been put to the test throughout this book. Unlearning what it means to be healthy will make it possible for you to explore options outside the medical industrial complex that can help you live the longest and healthiest life possible.

To gain the full benefits of your adaptability and defense system, you will need to protect your imagination from your own prejudices, from what you have already experienced or consider to be normal. You can accomplish this by arming yourself with two questions that will light a path toward new possibilities: "What if?" and "Why not?"

Wherever life takes you, you will be all right.

You are ready.

ACKNOWLEDGMENTS

This book was created to save lives. It was only made possible by the loving support and companionship of the extraordinary beings who surround us.

We would like to begin from the usual end, by first recognizing the two people who save our lives every day, Martha Garcia and Pasha Moshkalov. We thank them for being our sounding boards, wise guides, and most demanding critics. Their patience and persistence paid off.

We would like to thank our champions and co-conspirators, Seth Goldenberg and David Drake, for believing that our ideas about health should be shared widely.

We also would like to thank those accomplices who were willing to take risks and prove that health is much more than the absence of disease. Among the many who deserve to be mentioned here, we would like to single out Machteld Huber, Laura O'Grady, Fiona Godlee, Richard Smith, J André Knottnerus, Henk Smid, Murray Enkin, Sholom Glouberman, Howard Hu, Rani Kotha, Adriana Arango, Alejandro Gaviria, Mauricio Serra, and Nestor Rodriguez. We appreciate the courage and audacity it took to shake up the status quo. Invaluable insights were generated by the work of the Health of Humanity Project at the University of Toronto, which was made possible by the commitment of many people. It is worth mentioning Jenny Gatov, Andres Cabrera, Alberto Ruiz, Keiwan Wind, Farimah HakemZadeh, Angie Puerto, David Rodriguez, Sara Espinal, Svjetlana Kovacevic, and Ashita Mohapatra. Along the way, we were stimulated by the ideas of inspired thinkers, among whom Epictetus, Marcel Proust, Bertrand Russell, Ivan Illich, Roberto M. Unger, Lisa Feldman Barrett, Havi Carel, and Merlin Sheldrake stand out.

To our masterful editor, Madhulika Sikka, our immense gratitude for guiding us so kindly and effectively while nurturing this book. Each of her comments acted as a powerful invitation to take it to a higher level. We would also like to thank Aubrey Martinson for her editorial assistance and accompaniment throughout the process, and production editor Mark Birkey and copy editor Barbara Jatkola for their phenomenally conscientious and precise attention, which enlivened the music of our messages.

We now hope that this book will become a cherished companion to many people, who will revisit it often as they unleash their adapt-ability and stay healthy no matter what.

CHAPTER 1: WE GOT IT ALL WRONG

5 *"Health is a state"* Constitution of the World Health Organization. WHO; 1948. apps.who.int/gb/bd/pdf_files/BD_49th-en.pdf#page=6

5 *Just by having* Dental Caries (Tooth Decay) in Adults (Age 20 to 64). National Institute of Dental and Craniofacial Research. www.nidcr.nih.gov/research/data-statistics/dental-caries/adults

6 *An easy answer* Bickenbach J. WHO's definition of health: philosophical analysis. In: Schramme T, Edwards S, editors. *Handbook of the Philosophy of Medicine.* Springer Science+Business Media; 2015. pp. 1–14.

6 *Yet another possibility* Crawford R. Healthism and the medicalization of everyday life. *Int J Health Serv.* 1980;10(3):365–88.

6 *It would be known* Brundtland GH. The war against disease. *JAMA.* 2002 Jan 23;287(4):444.

6 *The motivation of humanity* Chan A. Penicillin: wonder drug of World War II. 2017. HistoryNet.com. historynet.com/penicillin-wonder-drug-world-war-ii.htm

6 *At that time* Roser M, Ortiz-Ospina E, Ritchie H. Life Expectancy. Our World in Data. 2013 May 23. ourworldindata.org/life-expectancy

6   *The allure of penicillin* Thom C. Mycology presents penicillin. *Mycologia*. 1945 Jul 1;37(4):460–75.

7   *By the time the WHO* Ballard K, Elston MA. Medicalisation: a multi-dimensional concept. *Soc Theory Health*. 2005 Aug 1; 3(3):228–41.

7   *As a consequence* Carter SK. Beyond control: body and self in women's childbearing narratives. *Sociol Health Illn*. 2010 Nov; 32(7):993–1009.

8   *Subsequently, many people* Zachar P, First MB, Kendler KS. The bereavement exclusion debate in the DSM-5: a history. *Clin Psychol Sci*. 2017 Sep 1;5(5):890–906.

8   *This expansion of medicine* Relman AS. The new medical-industrial complex. *N Engl J Med*. 1980 Oct 23;303(17):963–70.

8   *At the turn of the 21st century* Global Health Expenditure Database. World Health Organization. apps.who.int/nha/database/Select/Indicators/en

8   *and was feeding* Hunter BM, Murray SF. Deconstructing the financialization of healthcare. *Dev Change*. 2019 Sep 6;50(5): 1263–87.

8   *Today, the most advanced* Gmeinde M, Morgan D, Mueller M. How much do OECD countries spend on prevention? OECD Health Working Paper No. 101. Organisation for Economic Co-operation and Development. 2017 Dec 11. read.oecd-ilibrary .org/social-issues-migration-health/how-much-do-oecd-countries -spend-on-prevention_f19e803c-en

8   *The situation in the US* Papanicolas I, Woskie LR, Jha AK. Health care spending in the United States and other high-income countries. *JAMA*. 2018 Mar 13;319(10):1024–39.

9   *In the US, perhaps* Null G, Dean C, Feldman M, Rasio D, Smith D. Death by medicine. *J Orthomol Med*. 2005;20(1):21–34.
      Null G, Feldman M, Rasio D, Dean C. *Death by Medicine*. Axios Press; 2011.

10   *The invitation was* Jadad AR, O'Grady L. How should health be defined? *BMJ*. 2008 Dec 10;337:a2900.

10 *A global conversation* Jadad AR, O'Grady L. A global conversation on defining health. BMJ Opinion. *BMJ.* 2008 Dec 10. blogs .bmj.com/bmj/2008/12/10/alex-jadad-on-defining-health

11 *Taken all together* Huber M, Knottnerus JA, Green L, Horst H, Jadad AR, Kromhout D, et al. How should we define health? *BMJ.* 2011;343:d4163.

CHAPTER 2: HOW ARE YOU FEELING?

12 *By the late 1990s* Idler EL, Beyamini Y. Self-rated health and mortality: a review of twenty-seven community studies. *J Health Soc Behav.* 1997;38:21–37.

14 *This question has been used* Suchman EA, Phillips BS, Streib GF. An analysis of the validity of health questionnaires. *Soc Forces.* 1958;36(3):223–32.

14 *Physicians' power had* Waddington I. The movement towards the professionalization of medicine. *BMJ.* 1990 Oct 3;301(6754): 688–90.

14 *This had also* Illich I. Disabling professions. *ICC Quarterly.* 1978;5(1):23–32.

14 *Consequently, members* Caridi family, Poduri A, Devinsky O, Tabacinic M, Jadad AR. Experiencing positive health, as a family, while living with a rare complex disease: bringing participatory medicine through collaborative decision making into the real world. *J Particip Med.* 2020;12(2):e17602.

14 *This situation started* Eysenbach G, Jadad AR. Evidence-based patient choice and consumer health informatics in the internet age. *J Med Internet Res.* 2001 Apr;3(2):e19.
    Jadad AR. Promoting partnerships: challenges for the internet age. *BMJ.* 1999 Sep 18;319(7212):761–4.

15 *Negative self-assessed health* DeSalvo KB, Bloser N, Reynolds K, He J, Muntner P. Mortality prediction with a single general self-rated health question. *J Gen Intern Med.* 2006;21(3):267–75.
    Idler and Benyamini, Self-rated health and mortality.
    Ganna A, Ingelsson E. 5 year mortality predictors in 498 103

UK Biobank participants: a prospective population-based study. *Lancet.* 2015 Aug 8;386(9993):533–40.

Jylhä M. What is self-rated health and why does it predict mortality? Towards a unified conceptual model. *Soc Sci Med.* 2009 Aug;69(3):307–16.

15 *You are also more likely to* Lee Y. The predictive value of self assessed general, physical, and mental health on functional decline and mortality in older adults. *J Epidemiol Community Health* 2000;54(2):123–9.

Lee HY, Kim J, Merighi JR. Physical activity and self-rated health status among older adult cancer survivors: does intensity of activity play a role? *Oncol Nurs Forum.* 2015 Nov;42(6): 614–24.

Johar M, Jones G, Savage E. The effect of lifestyle choices on emergency department use in Australia. *Health Policy.* 2013 May;110(2–3):280–90.

Huohvanainen E, Strandberg AY, Stenholm S, Pitkälä KH, Tilvis RS, Strandberg TE. Association of self-rated health in midlife with mortality and old age frailty: a 26-year follow-up of initially healthy men. *J Gerontol A Biol Sci Med Sci.* 2016 Jul;71(7):923–8.

Mavaddat N, Parker RA, Sanderson S, Mant J, Kinmonth AL. Relationship of self-rated health with fatal and non-fatal outcomes in cardiovascular disease: a systematic review and meta-analysis. *PLoS One.* 2014 Jul 30;9(7):e103509.

15 *What is even more* Cho H, Wang Z, Yabroff KR, Liu B, McNeel T, Feuer EJ, et al. Estimating life expectancy adjusted by self-rated health status in the United States: national health interview survey linked to the mortality. *BMC Public Health.* 2022; 22:141.

15 *Those with advanced cancer* Shadbolt B, Barresi J, Craft P. Self-rated health as a predictor of survival among patients with advanced cancer. *J Clin Oncol.* 2002 May 15;20(10):2514–9.

16 *They show how well* Kananen L, Enroth L, Raitanen J, Jylhävä J, Bürkle A, Moreno-Villanueva M, et al. Self-rated health in individuals with and without disease is associated with multiple bio-

markers representing multiple biological domains. *Sci Rep.* 2021 Mar 17;11(1):6139.

16 *For example, in the US* Centers for Disease Control and Prevention. Racial/ethnic disparities in self-rated health status among adults with and without disabilities—United States, 2004–2006. *MMWR Morb Mortal Wkly Rep.* 2008 Oct 3;57(39):1069–73.

17 *To provide some context* Boersma P, Black LI, Ward BW. Prevalence of multiple chronic conditions among US adults, 2018. *Prev Chronic Dis.* 2020 Sep 17;17:e106.

17 *Data from Canada* Bamia C, Orfanos P, Juerges H, Schöttker B, Brenner H, Lorbeer R, et al. Self-rated health and all-cause and cause-specific mortality of older adults: individual data meta-analysis of prospective cohort studies in the CHANCES consortium. *Maturitas.* 2017 Sep;103:37–44.

Nützel A, Dahlhaus A, Fuchs A, Gensichen J, König H-H, Riedel-Heller S, et al. Self-rated health in multimorbid older general practice patients: a cross-sectional study in Germany. *BMC Fam Pract.* 2014 Jan 3;15:1.

Northwood M, Ploeg J, Markle-Reid M, Sherifali D. Integrative review of the social determinants of health in older adults with multimorbidity. *J Adv Nurs.* 2017 Aug 3 ;74(1):45–60. dx.doi.org /10.1111/jan.13408

Barnett K, Mercer SW, Norbury M, Watt G, Wyke S, Guthrie B. Epidemiology of multimorbidity and implications for health care, research, and medical education: a cross-sectional study. *Lancet.* 2012 Jul 7;380(9836):37–43.

17 *The figure remains above* Terner et al., Chronic conditions more than age drive health system use.

17 *Furthermore, a study* Shadbolt et al., Self-rated health as a predictor of survival.

18 *What was also consistent* Jylhä, What is self-rated health?

Tissue T. Another look at self-rated health among the elderly. *J Gerontol.* 1972 Jan;27(1):91–4.

Mackenbach JP, Simon JG, Looman CWN, Joung IMA. Self-assessed health and mortality: could psychosocial factors explain the association? *Int J Epidemiol.* 2002 Dec;31(6):1162–8.

Suls J, Marco CA, Tobin S. The role of temporal comparison, social comparison, and direct appraisal in the elderly's self-evaluations of health. *J Appl Soc Psychol.* 1991 Jul;21(14): 1125–44.

18   *We found that* Jadad AR, Arango A, Sepúlveda JD, Espinal S, Rodríguez D, Wind K, editors. *Unleashing a Pandemic of Health from the Workplace: Believing Is Seeing.* Beati; 2017.

18   *men tend to report* Jylhä M, Guralnik JM, Ferrucci L, Jokela J, Heikkinen E. Is self-rated health comparable across cultures and genders? *J Gerontol B Psychol Sci Soc Sci.* 1998 May;53(3): s144–52.

Franks P, Gold MR, Fiscella K. Sociodemographics, self-rated health, and mortality in the US. *Soc Sci Med.* 2003 Jun;56(12): 2505–14.

18   *Men are also more likely* Undén A-L, Elofsson S. Do different factors explain self-rated health in men and women? *Gend Med.* 2006 Dec;3(4):295–308.

19   *Older people* Jylhä, What is self-rated health?

Simon JG, De Boer JB, Joung IMA, Bosma H, Mackenbach JP. How is your health in general? A qualitative study on self-assessed health. *Eur J Public Health.* 2005 Apr;15(2):200–8.

19   *They presented us with* Serra M, Palacio DO, Espinal S, Rodriguez DG, Jadad AR. *Trusted Networks: The Key to Achieve World-Class Health Outcomes on a Shoestring.* Beati; 2018.

21   *To figure this out* Espinosa NG, Añez M, Serra M, Espinal S, Rodriguez DG, Jadad AR, editors. *Toward Sustainable Well-Being for All.* Beati; 2020.

22   *These high levels* Rytter D, Rask CU, Vestergaard CH, Nybo Andersen A-M, Bech BH. Non-specific health complaints and self-rated health in pre-adolescents: impact on primary health care use. *Sci Rep.* 2020 Feb 24;10(1):3292.

CHAPTER 3: ADAPT-ABILITY

24   *In the 1970s* Antonovsky A, Maoz B, Dowty N, Wijsenbeek H. Twenty-five years later: a limited study of the sequelae of the

concentration camp experience. *Soc Psychiatry*. 1971 Dec;6(4): 186–93.

25 ***And yet, when probed*** Torr BM, Walsh ET. Does the refugee experience overshadow the effect of SES? An examination of self-reported health among older Vietnamese refugees. *Race Soc Probl.* 2018 Sep 1;10(3):259–71.

25 ***Despite the hardship*** Lee JW. The effect of income on health after Hurricane Katrina. PhD dissertation. City University of New York. 2014. academicworks.cuny.edu/cgi/viewcontent.cgi?referer =&httpsredir=1&article=1503&context=gc_etds

26 ***Research in France showed*** Recchi E, Ferragina E, Helmeid E, Pauly S, Safi M, Sauger N, et al. The "eye of the hurricane" paradox: an unexpected and unequal rise of well-being during the Covid-19 lockdown in France. *Res Soc Stratif Mobil.* 2020 Aug;68:100508.

26 ***This unusual phenomenon*** Peters A, Rospleszcz S, Greiser KH, Dallavalle M, Berger K, et al. The impact of the COVID-19 pandemic on self-reported health. *Dtsch Arztebl Int.* 2020 Dec 11;117(50):861–7.

26 ***In essence, adaptability*** Vaillant GE. *Adaptation to Life.* Harvard University Press; 1977.

   Martin AJ. Adaptability and learning. In: Seel NM, editor. *Encyclopedia of the Sciences of Learning.* Springer US; 2012. pp. 90–92.

   Hollis KL. Adaptation and learning. In: Seel NM, editor. *Encyclopedia of the Sciences of Learning.* Springer US; 2012. pp. 95–8.

27 ***To a large extent*** Gopnik A. *The Gardener and the Carpenter.* Farrar, Straus and Giroux; 2016.

27 ***Childhood can, therefore*** Gopnik A. *The Philosophical Baby.* Farrar, Straus and Giroux; 2009.

27 ***With this, it becomes*** Fischer MD. Cultural agents: a community of minds. In: Dikenelli O, Gleizes MP, Ricci A, editors. *Engineering Societies in the Agents World VI.* Springer Berlin Heidelberg; 2006. pp. 259–74.

28 *This has given rise* Pagel M. Evolution: adapted to culture. *Nature.* 2012 Feb 15;482(7385):297–9.

28 *Cultures can also enable* Whiten A, Hinde RA, Laland KN, Stringer CB. Culture evolves. *Philos Trans R Soc Lond B Biol Sci.* 2011 Apr 12;366(1567):938–48.

29 *These processes include* Modell H, Cliff W, Michael J, McFarland J, Wenderoth MP, Wright A. A physiologist's view of homeostasis. *Adv Physiol Educ.* 2015 Dec;39(4):259–66.

29 *Its main goal is* Kleckner IR, Zhang J, Touroutoglou A, Chanes L, Xia C, Simmons WK, et al. Evidence for a large-scale brain system supporting allostasis and interoception in humans. *Nat Hum Behav.* 2017 Apr 24;1:0069. dx.doi.org/10.1038/s41562-017-0069

29 *Even though the water* Barrett LF. *Seven and a Half Lessons About the Brain.* Houghton Mifflin Harcourt; 2020.

30 *The brain, as a prediction* Tsakiris M, Critchley H. Interoception beyond homeostasis: affect, cognition and mental health. *Philos Trans R Soc Lond B Biol Sci.* 2016 Nov 19;371(1708):20160002.

30 *In this way, interoception* Quigley KS, Kanoski S, Grill WM, Barrett LF, Tsakiris M. Functions of interoception: from energy regulation to experience of the self. *Trends Neurosci.* 2021 Jan;44(1):29–38.

Jylhä M. What is self-rated health and why does it predict mortality? Towards a unified conceptual model. *Soc Sci Med.* 2009 Aug;69(3):307–16.

31 *For instance, people* Handschu R, Poppe R, Rauss J, Neundörfer B, Erbguth F. Emergency calls in acute stroke. *Stroke.* 2003 Apr;34(4):1005–9.

32 *Humor is a wonderful* Villeneuve A. Why paramedics go for the punch(line). *Dartmouth Medicine.* Spring 2005. dartmed.dartmouth.edu/spring05/html/disc_paramedics.php

Christopher S. An introduction to black humour as a coping mechanism for student paramedics. *JPP.* 2015 Dec 2;7(12):610–7.

32 *The value of humor* Christie W, Moore C. The impact of humor on patients with cancer. *Clin J Oncol Nurs.* 2005 Apr;9(2):211–8.

33 *Research has shown* Temel JS, Greer JA, Muzikansky A, Galla-
gher ER, Admane S, Jackson VA, et al. Early palliative care for
patients with metastatic non-small-cell lung cancer. *N Engl J Med.*
2010 Aug 19;363(8):733–42.

CHAPTER 4: THE TOXIC STRESS LOAD

36 *A baby born* Schencker L. Chicago's lifespan gap: Streeterville
residents live to 90. Englewood residents die at 60. Study finds
it's the largest divide in the U.S. *Chicago Tribune.* 2019 Jun 5.
chicagotribune.com/business/ct-biz-chicago-has-largest-life
-expectancy-gap-between-neighborhoods-20190605-story.html

36 *The same study showed* Large life expectancy gaps in U.S. cities
linked to racial and ethnic segregation by neighborhood. NYC
Langone Health. 2009 Jun 5. nyulangone.org/news/large-life
-expectancy-gaps-us-cities-linked-racial-ethnic-segregation
-neighborhood
        Ducharme J, Wolfson E. Your ZIP code might determine how
long you live—and the difference could be decades. *Time.* 2019
Jun 17. time.com/5608268/zip-code-health

36 *At the time* Life expectancy at birth, total (years). World Bank.
data.worldbank.org/indicator/SP.DYN.LE00.IN

37 *This is the physical* Shern DL, Blanch AK, Steverman SM. Impact of toxic stress on individuals and communities: a review of
the literature. Report. Mental Health America. 2014. mhanational
.org/sites/default/files/Impact%20of%20Toxic%20Stress%20
on%20Individuals%20and%20Communities-A%20Review%20
of%20the%20Literature.pdf

37 *The second is* McEwen BS, Stellar E. Stress and the individual:
mechanisms leading to disease. *Arch Intern Med.* 1993 Sep
27;153(18):2093–101.

37 *It can also lead* Lewis TT, Cogburn CD, Williams DR. Self-
reported experiences of discrimination and health: scientific advances, ongoing controversies, and emerging issues. *Annu Rev
Clin Psychol.* 2015 Jan 2;11:407–40.
        Guidi J, Lucente M, Sonino N, Fava GA. Allostatic load and

its impact on health: a systematic review. *Psychother Psychosom.* 2021;90(1):11–27.

37 **Such changes are so profound** Geronimus AT, Hicken M, Keene D, Bound J. "Weathering" and age patterns of allostatic load scores among Blacks and Whites in the United States. *Am J Public Health.* 2006 May 1;96(5):826–33.

Forde AT, Crookes DM, Suglia SF, Demmer RT. The weathering hypothesis as an explanation for racial disparities in health: a systematic review. *Ann Epidemiol.* 2019 May;33:1–18.e3.

37 **Adding insult to injury** Suvarna B, Suvarna A, Phillips R, Juster R-P, McDermott B, Sarnyai Z. Health risk behaviours and allostatic load: a systematic review. *Neurosci Biobehav Rev.* 2020 Jan;108:694–711.

37 **Such behaviors feed** Williams DR, Lawrence JA, Davis BA. Racism and health: evidence and needed research. *Annu Rev Public Health.* 2019 Apr 1;40:105–25.

Paradies Y, Ben J, Denson N, Elias A, Priest N, Pieterse A, et al. Racism as a determinant of health: a systematic review and meta-analysis. *PLoS One.* 2015 Sep 23;10(9):e0138511.

38 **It can even** Golding J, Gregory S, Northstone K, Pembrey M, Watkins S, Iles-Caven Y, et al. Human transgenerational observations of regular smoking before puberty on fat mass in grandchildren and great-grandchildren. *Sci Rep.* 2022;12:1139. nature .com/articles/s41598-021-04504-0

38 **As a result, burnout** Hill A. A brief history of executive burnout. *Financial Times.* 2019 Jun 5. ft.com/content/84a0f3b8-76f4 -11e9-b0ec-7dff87b9a4a2

38 **Such pressures often push** Roderick M, Allen-Collinson J. "I just want to be left alone": novel sociological insights into dramaturgical demands on professional athletes. *Sociol Sport J.* 2020 Mar 9;37(2):108–16.

38 **In some cases, they maladapt** Rockwell D, Giles DC. Being a celebrity: a phenomenology of fame. *J Phenomenol Psychol.* 2009;40(2):178.

Misra N, Srivastava S. The fallacy of happiness: a psychological investigation of suicide among successful people. In: Motta R, editor. *Suicide*. IntechOpen; 2021.

39   ***Often, this mounting TSL*** Rockwell and Giles, Being a celebrity.

39   ***This label began*** Zinn H. *A People's History of the United States*. Routledge; 2015.

39   ***This practice came into conflict*** Omi M, Winant H. *Racial Formation in the United States*. Routledge; 2014.

39   ***This allowed for*** Fredrickson GM. *Racism: A Short History*. Princeton University Press; 2015.

40   ***Even though the existence*** Kolbert E. There's no scientific basis for race—it's a made-up label. *National Geographic*. 2018 Mar 12. nationalgeographic.com/magazine/article/race-genetics-science -africa

Loveman M. *National Colors: Racial Classification and the State in Latin America*. Oxford University Press; 2014.

Brubaker R. Ethnicity, race, and nationalism. *Annu Rev Sociol*. 2009 Jul 6. annualreviews.org/doi/abs/10.1146/annurev-soc -070308-115916

McNamee L. Colonial legacies and comparative racial identification in the Americas. *Am J Sociol*. 2020 Sep 1;126(2):318–53.

40   ***This sorting has created*** Timberlake JM, Ignatov, MD. Residential segregation. Oxford Bibliographies. 2019. oxfordbibliog raphies.com/view/document/obo-9780199756384/obo -9780199756384-0116.xml

40   ***Once segregation occurs*** The root causes of health inequity. In: Weinstein JN, Geller A, Negussie Y, Baciu A, editors. *Communities in Action: Pathways to Health Equity*. National Academies Press; 2017.

40   ***In the Englewood neighborhood*** Fredrick E. Death, violence, health, and poverty in Chicago. *Harvard Health Policy Rev*. 2018;19:1–25.

40   ***Meanwhile, in Streeterville*** Streeterville neighborhood in Chicago, Illinois (IL), 60611 detailed profile. City-Data.com. city -data.com/neighborhood/Streeterville-Chicago-IL.html

40 **Higher rates of premature death** Anderson KF, Simburger D. Racial/ethnic residential segregation, poor self-rated health, and the moderating role of immigration. *Race Soc Probl.* 2021 Jul 23. link.springer.com/10.1007/s12552-021-09345-0

40 **the mortality rate associated with** Soth A. Only eight miles apart, the Streeterville and Englewood neighborhoods of Chicago have a life-expectancy gap of roughly 30 years. *New York Times.* 2020 Sep 5. nytimes.com/interactive/2020/09/05/opinion/inequality-life-expectancy.html

40 **This emerging pattern** Siegel M, Critchfield-Jain I, Boykin M, Owens A. Actual racial/ethnic disparities in COVID-19 mortality for the non-Hispanic Black compared to non-Hispanic White population in 35 US states and their association with structural racism. *J Racial Ethn Health Disparities.* 2021 Apr 27. doi .org/10.1007/s40615-021-01028-1

40 **This underscores the insight** Iton A, Ross RK. Understanding how health happens: your zip code is more important than your genetic code. In: Callahan R, Bhattachanya D, editors. *Public Health Leadership.* Routledge; 2017. pp. 83–99.

41 **When the list is viewed** Life expectancy at birth.

41 **How much of this** Bell CN, Thorpe RJ Jr, LaVeist TA. The role of social context in racial disparities in self-rated health. *J Urban Health.* 2018 Feb;95(1):13–20.

41 **What makes ethnicity** Eriksen TH. Ethnicity. In: Eriksen TH, editor. The Wiley-Blackwell Encyclopedia of Globalization; Wiley; 2012 Feb 29. onlinelibrary.wiley.com/doi/10.1002/9780470670590.wbeog179

Peoples J, Bailey G. *Humanity: An Introduction to Cultural Anthropology.* Cengage Learning; 2017.

42 **The data on this group** Vidal-Ortiz S, Martínez J. Latinx thoughts: Latinidad with an X. *Lat Stud.* 2018 Oct 1;16(3): 384–95.

Chen D. Implicit racial/ethnic bias and Latino health: a systematic review. Thesis. Arizona State University. 2017. repository .asu.edu/items/45647

42   ***They are also victims*** Tessler RA, Langton L, Rivara FP, Vavilala MS, Rowhani-Rahbar A. Differences by victim race and ethnicity in race- and ethnicity-motivated violent bias crimes: a national study. *J Interpers Violence.* 2021 Jul;36(13–14):6297–318.

      Anderson and Simburger, Racial/ethnic residential segregation.

42   ***A more interesting alternative*** Llabre MM. Insight into the Hispanic paradox: the language hypothesis. *Perspect Psychol Sci.* 2021 Feb 23;16(6):1324–36.

43   ***Lastly, it has been suggested*** Ruiz JM, Steffen P, Smith TB. Hispanic mortality paradox: a systematic review and meta-analysis of the longitudinal literature. *Am J Public Health.* 2013 Mar;103(3): e52–60.

43   ***Although the idea*** Pines G. The contentious history of the passport. *National Geographic.* 2017 May 16. nationalgeographic .com/travel/article/a-history-of-the-passport

43   ***Their entry was restricted*** Markel H, Stern AM. The foreignness of germs: the persistent association of immigrants and disease in American society. *Milbank Q.* 2002;80(4):757–88.

43   ***How could immigrants' origins*** Pines, Contentious history of the passport.

43   ***In fact, recent immigrants*** Argeseanu Cunningham S, Ruben JD, Narayan KMV. Health of foreign-born people in the United States: a review. *Health Place.* 2008 Dec;14(4):623–35.

44   ***Over time, a change*** Ng E. The healthy immigrant effect and mortality rates. *Health Rep.* 2011 Dec;22(4):25–9.

44   ***In the end*** Berry JW. Contexts of acculturation. In: Sam DL, Berry JW, editors. *The Cambridge Handbook of Acculturation Psychology.* Cambridge University Press; 2006. pp. 27–42.

44   ***These consequences are*** Scholaske L, Wadhwa PD, Entringer S. Acculturation and biological stress markers: a systematic review. *Psychoneuroendocrinology.* 2021 Jul 1;132:105349.

44   ***Another label*** Marmot MG. Status syndrome: a challenge to medicine. *JAMA.* 2006 Mar 15;295(11):1304–7.

45   *A study of Oscar-winning actors* Redelmeier DA, Singh SM. Survival in Academy Award–winning actors and actresses. *Ann Intern Med.* 2001 May 15;134(10):955–62.

     Redelmeier DA, Singh SM. Longevity of screenwriters who win an Academy Award: longitudinal study. *BMJ.* 2001; 323(7327):1491–6.

45   *Something similar is found* Marmot M. The health gap: the challenge of an unequal world. *Lancet.* 2015 Dec 12;386(10011): 2442–4.

46   *From the biological perspective* McCarthy MM. Stress during pregnancy: fetal males pay the price. *Proc Natl Acad Sci U S A.* 2019 Nov 26;116(48):23877–9.

46   *In fact, the male* Zhao D, Zou L, Lei X, Zhang Y. Gender differences in infant mortality and neonatal morbidity in mixed-gender twins. *Sci Rep.* 2017 Aug 18;7(1):8736.

46   *Some of the explanations* Marais GAB, Gaillard J-M, Vieira C, Plotton I, Sanlaville D, Gueyffier F, et al. Sex gap in aging and longevity: can sex chromosomes play a role? *Biol Sex Differ.* 2018 Jul 17;9(1):33.

     Hägg S, Jylhävä J. Sex differences in biological aging with a focus on human studies. *eLife.* 2021 May 13;10. dx.doi.org/10.7554/eLife.63425

46   *Other studies suggest* Regan JC, Partridge L. Gender and longevity: why do men die earlier than women? Comparative and experimental evidence. *Best Pract Res Clin Endocrinol Metab.* 2013 Aug;27(4):467–79.

46   *This hormonal difference* Bouman A, Heineman MJ, Faas MM. Sex hormones and the immune response in humans. *Hum Reprod Update.* 2005 Jul;11(4):411–23.

46   *These natural advantages* Austad SN, Fischer KE. Sex differences in lifespan. *Cell Metab.* 2016 Jun 14;23(6):1022–33.

     Lemaître J-F, Ronget V, Tidière M, Allainé D, Berger V, Cohas A, et al. Sex differences in adult lifespan and aging rates of mortality across wild mammals. *Proc Natl Acad Sci U S A.* 2020 Apr 14;117(15):8546–53.

46 *An increased TSL* Sundberg L, Agahi N, Fritzell J, Fors S. Why is the gender gap in life expectancy decreasing? The impact of age- and cause-specific mortality in Sweden 1997–2014. *Int J Public Health.* 2018 Jul 1;63(6):673–81.

46 *This started to happen* Zarulli V, Kashnitsky I, Vaupel JW. Death rates at specific life stages mold the sex gap in life expectancy. *Proc Natl Acad Sci U S A.* 2021 May 18;118(20). dx.doi.org/10.1073/pnas.2010588118

Annandale E. Health and gender. In: Cockerham WC, editor. *The Wiley Blackwell Companion to Medical Sociology.* Wiley-Blackwell; 2021. pp. 237–57.

47 *Even though females* Luy M, Minagawa Y. Gender gaps—life expectancy and proportion of life in poor health. *Health Rep.* 2014 Dec;25(12):12–9.

47 *This conundrum was* Oksuzyan A, Petersen I, Stovring H, Bingley P, Vaupel JW, Christensen K. The male-female health-survival paradox: a survey and register study of the impact of sex-specific selection and information bias. *Ann Epidemiol.* 2009 Jul 1;19(7):504–11.

47 *In other words* Luy and Minagawa, Gender gaps.

47 *An ethnic minority female* Compare the Two Speeches. Sojourner Truth Project. thesojournertruthproject.com/compare-the-speeches

47 *This "simultaneity" of labels* Smith B. Some home truths on the contemporary black feminist movement. *Black Scholar.* 1985; 16(2):4–13.

48 *It became a core framework* Crenshaw K. Demarginalizing the intersection of race and sex: a black feminist critique of antidiscrimination doctrine, feminist theory and antiracist politics. *Univ Chic Leg Forum.* 1989;139.

48 *This led to the recognition* Haeberer M, León-Gómez I, Pérez-Gómez B, Tellez-Plaza M, Rodríguez-Artalejo F, Galán I. Social inequalities in cardiovascular mortality in Spain from an intersectional perspective. *Rev Esp Cardiol.* 2020 Apr;73(4):282–9.

Cummings JL, Braboy Jackson P. Race, gender, and SES disparities in self-assessed health, 1974–2004. *Res Aging*. 2008 Mar 1;30(2):137–67.

48 **Death by suicide among physicians** Harvey SB, Epstein RM, Glozier N, Petrie K, Strudwick J, Gayed A, et al. Mental illness and suicide among physicians. *Lancet*. 2021 Sep 4;398(10303): 920–30.

Duarte D, El-Hagrassy MM, Couto TCE, Gurgel W, Fregni F, Correa H. Male and female physician suicidality: a systematic review and meta-analysis. *JAMA Psychiatry*. 2020 Jun 1;77(6): 587–97.

Ye GY, Davidson JE, Kim K, Zisook S. Physician death by suicide in the United States: 2012–2016. *J Psychiatr Res*. 2021 Feb 1;134:158–65.

Petrie K, Crawford J, Baker STE, Dean K, Robinson J, Veness BG, et al. Interventions to reduce symptoms of common mental disorders and suicidal ideation in physicians: a systematic review and meta-analysis. *Lancet Psychiatry*. 2019 Mar;6(3): 225–34.

49 **However, they fare better** Zhang L, Bo A, Lu W. To unfold the immigrant paradox: maltreatment risk and mental health of racial-ethnic minority children. *Front Public Health*. 2021 Feb 17;9:619164.

49 **Another conundrum is** Hainer V, Aldhoon-Hainerová I. Obesity paradox does exist. *Diabetes Care*. 2013 Aug;36 (Suppl 2): S276–81.

49 **These paradoxes suggest** Robards F, Kang M, Luscombe G, Hawke C, Sanci L, Steinbeck K, et al. Intersectionality: social marginalisation and self-reported health status in young people. *Int J Environ Res Public Health*. 2020 Nov 3;17(21). dx.doi .org/10.3390/ijerph17218104

Roxo L, Bambra C, Perelman J. Gender equality and gender inequalities in self-reported health: a longitudinal study of 27 European countries 2004 to 2016. *Int J Health Serv*. 2021 Apr; 51(2):146–54.

49 **Therefore, the group** Global passport power rank 2021. Passport Index. passportindex.org/passport-power-rank-2021.php

50   *At the time* Central Intelligence Agency. Explore all coun-
      tries: Monaco. The World Factbook. cia.gov/the-world-factbook/
      countries/monaco

      Intentional homicides (per 100,000 people)—Monaco. World
      Bank. data.worldbank.org/indicator/VC.IHR.PSRC.P5?locations
      =MC&most_recent_value_desc=true

50   *The per capita income* Warren K. I spent 5 days in Monaco.
      Here's what life looks like in a land so wealthy it doesn't even track
      poverty rates. *Business Insider.* 2019 Dec 24. businessinsider.com/
      monaco-wealth-poverty-life-photos-2019-11

50   *These are regions* Buettner D, Skemp S. Blue Zones: lessons from
      the world's longest lived. *Am J Lifestyle Med.* 2016 Sep;10(5):
      318–21.

50   *Aside from being isolated* Buettner D. Power 9°: Reverse engi-
      neering longevity. Blue Zones. 2016. bluezones.com/2016/11/
      power-9

50   *Studies on centenarians* Newman SJ. Supercentenarians and the
      oldest-old are concentrated into regions with no birth certificates
      and short lifespans. bioRxiv. 2021. link.springer.com/content/
      pdf/10.1007%2F978-3-642-11520-2.pdf

51   *Then, between the 1950s* Vaupel JW, Jeune B. The emergence and
      proliferation of centenarians. In: Jeune B, Vaupel JW, editors. *Ex-
      ceptional Longevity: From Prehistory to the Present.* Odense Uni-
      versity Press; 1994. pp. 1–14. Monographs on Population Aging 2.

51   *Assuming that the pace* Christensen K, Doblhammer G, Rau R,
      Vaupel JW. Ageing populations: the challenges ahead. *Lancet.*
      2009 Oct 3;374(9696):1196–208.

51   *Another interesting insight* Fries JF, Nesse RM, Schneider EL.
      Aging, natural death, and the compression of morbidity. *N Engl J
      Med.* 1984 Mar 8;310(10):659–60.

51   *Rather than escaping* Borras C, Ingles M, Mas-Bargues C, Drom-
      ant M, Sanz-Ros J, Román-Domínguez A, et al. Centenarians: an
      excellent example of resilience for successful ageing. *Mech Ageing
      Dev.* 2020 Mar;186:111199.

51   *Although they appear* Hagberg B, Samuelsson G. Survival after
     100 years of age: a multivariate model of exceptional survival in
     Swedish centenarians. *J Gerontol A Biol Sci Med Sci.* 2008
     Nov;63(11):1219–26.
          Alvarez J-A, Medford A, Strozza C, Thinggaard M, Chris-
     tensen K. Stratification in health and survival after age 100:
     evidence from Danish centenarians. *BMC Geriatr.* 2021 Jul 1;
     21(1):406.

51   *These characteristics include* Pignolo RJ. Exceptional human
     longevity. *Mayo Clin Proc.* 2019 Jan 1;94(1):110–24.

52   *A team that* Gerontology Research Group. Gerontology Wiki.
     gerontology.wikia.org/wiki/Gerontology_Research_Group
          Santos-Lozano A, Sanchis-Gomar F, Pareja-Galeano H, Fiuza-
     Luces C, Emanuele E, Lucia A, et al. Where are supercentenarians
     located? A worldwide demographic study. *Rejuvenation Res.*
     2015 Feb;18(1):14–9.

52   *The longest-lived humans* Supercentenarians landscape overview.
     Report. Ageing Analytics Agency and Gerontology Research
     Group. 2020. data.longevity.international/Supercentenarians
     -Landscape-Overview-Report.pdf

52   *In our society's pursuit of* Olshansky SJ. From lifespan to health-
     span. *JAMA.* 2018 Oct 2;320(13):1323–4.

52   *By changing their thresholds* Pinquart M. Correlates of subjec-
     tive health in older adults: a meta-analysis. *Psychol Aging.*
     2001;16(3):414–26.

52   *Even obesity in this group* Tigani X, Artemiadis AK, Alexopou-
     los EC, Chrousos GP, Darviri C. Self-rated health in centenari-
     ans: a nation-wide cross-sectional Greek study. *Arch Gerontol
     Geriatr.* 2012 May;54(3):e342–8.

53   *Those who live the longest* Poon LW, Martin P, Bishop A, Cho J,
     da Rosa G, Deshpande N, et al. Understanding centenarians' psy-
     chosocial dynamics and their contributions to health and quality
     of life. *Curr Gerontol Geriatr Res.* 2010 Sep 26. dx.doi.org/10
     .1155/2010/680657

CHAPTER 5: YOU ARE WHAT YOU THINK

55   *A 2019 survey of adults* Survey reveals tension between financial stress and optimistic financial outlook among U.S. consumers. CreditWise from Capital One. 2019. prnewswire.com/news -releases/survey-reveals-tension-between-financial-stress-and -optimistic-financial-outlook-among-us-consumers-300940048 .html

55   *In 2020, other surveys* Mind over money study: getting in the right money mindset. Capital One and The Decision Lab. 2020. capitalone.com/about/newsroom/2020-capitalone -mindovermoneystudytips
        Thriving wallet: research insights report/white paper. Discover and Thrive Global. 2020. content.thriveglobal.com/wp -content/uploads/2020/02/Thriving-Wallet-Research-Insights -Report.pdf

55   *Indeed, financial concerns* BlackRock Global Investor Pulse: the world's largest study on the relationship between wealth and well-being. BlackRock. 2019. blackrock.com/corporate/insights/ investor-pulse
        Stress in America: paying with our health. Report. American Psychological Association. 2015. apa.org/news/press/releases/ stress/2014/stress-report.pdf

55   *Americans attribute their* Freeman G. AmOne.Com survey: consumers reveal their biggest financial fear. AmOne. 2019. investor.quinstreet.com/static-files/ead04c61-e8e2-4874-b24c -ef85a72bcdb6

56   *Technically speaking* Anxiety. APA Dictionary of Psychology. Accessed 2022 Apr 27. dictionary.apa.org/anxiety
        LaBar KS. Fear and anxiety. In: Feldman Barrett L, Lewis M, Haviland-Jones JM, editors. *Handbook of Emotions.* Guilford Press; 2016. pp. 751–73.

56   *Such episodes typically include* Anxiety disorders. Mayo Clinic. mayoclinic.org/diseases-conditions/anxiety/symptoms-causes /syc-20350961

56   *The money worries* De Nardi M, French E, Jones JB. Life expectancy and old age savings. NBER Working Paper No. 14653. Na-

tional Bureau of Economic Research. 2009 Jan. nber.org/papers/w14653

56 *You would experience fear* Bracha HS, Ralston TC, Matsukawa JM, Williams AE, Bracha DS. Does "fight or flight" need updating? *Psychosomatics.* 2004;45:448–9.

57 *Anxiety is very different* Richardson T, Elliott P, Roberts R. The relationship between personal unsecured debt and mental and physical health: a systematic review and meta-analysis. *Clin Psychol Rev.* 2013 Dec;33(8):1148–62.

57 *When this happens* Remes O, Brayne C, Van der Linde R, Lafortune L. A systematic review of reviews on the prevalence of anxiety disorders in adult populations. *Brain Behav.* 2016 Jul;6(7): e00497.

58 *The frequency of anxiety disorders* Baxter AJ, Scott KM, Vos T, Whiteford HA. Global prevalence of anxiety disorders: a systematic review and meta-regression. *Psychol Med.* 2013 May;43(5): 897–910.

58 *Regardless of culture* Baxter AJ, Scott KM, Ferrari AJ, Norman RE, Vos T, Whiteford HA. Challenging the myth of an "epidemic" of common mental disorders: trends in the global prevalence of anxiety and depression between 1990 and 2010. *Depress Anxiety.* 2014 Jun;31(6):506–16.

58 *Anxiety disorders are* Remes et al. A systematic review of reviews.

58 *In half of the cases* Regier DA, Rae DS, Narrow WE, Kaelber CT, Schatzberg AF. Prevalence of anxiety disorders and their comorbidity with mood and addictive disorders. *Br J Psychiatry.* 1998;(Suppl 34):24–8.

58 *Given the large number* Weisberg RB, Gonsalves MA, Ramadurai R, Braham H, Fuchs C, Beard C. Development of a cognitive bias modification intervention for anxiety disorders in primary care. *Br J Clin Psychol.* 2021 Feb 25.

Weisberg RB, Beard C, Moitra E, Dyck I, Keller MB. Adequacy of treatment received by primary care patients with anxiety disorders. *Depress Anxiety.* 2014 May;31(5):443–50.

58 *Of those, the vast majority* Parker EL, Banfield M, Fassnacht DB, Hatfield T, Kyrios M. Contemporary treatment of anxiety in pri-

mary care: a systematic review and meta-analysis of outcomes in countries with universal healthcare. *BMC Fam Pract.* 2021 May 15;22(1):92.

58 ***There is no such thing*** Ledoux J. *The Emotional Brain: The Mysterious Underpinnings of Emotional Life.* Simon and Schuster; 1998.

Tovote P, Fadok JP, Lüthi A. Neuronal circuits for fear and anxiety. *Nat Rev Neurosci.* 2015 Jun;16(6):317–31.

Méndez-Bértolo C, Moratti S, Toledano R, Lopez-Sosa F, Martínez-Alvarez R, Mah YH, et al. A fast pathway for fear in human amygdala. *Nat Neurosci.* 2016 Aug;19(8):1041–9.

Edwards SP. The amygdala: the body's alarm circuit. Brain-Work. The Dana Foundation. 2005. dnalc.cshl.edu/view/822 -The-Amygdala-the-Body-s-Alarm-Circuit.html

58 ***In fact, emotions*** Feldman Barrett L. *How Emotions Are Made.* Pan Macmillan; 2017.

59 ***It prepares the body*** McNaughton N, Corr PJ. A two-dimensional neuropsychology of defense: fear/anxiety and defensive distance. *Neurosci Biobehav Rev.* 2004 May;28(3):285–305.

60 ***In this way, you can view*** Barrett B, Zepeda E, Pollack L, Munson A, Sih A. Counter-culture: does social learning help or hinder adaptive response to human-induced rapid environmental change? *Front Ecol Evol.* 2019;7:183.

61 ***One of the most promising*** Beard C. Cognitive bias modification for anxiety: current evidence and future directions. *Expert Rev Neurother.* 2011 Feb;11(2):299–311.

Kahneman D. *Thinking, Fast and Slow.* 1st ed. Farrar, Straus and Giroux; 2011.

61 ***Attention bias is the tendency*** Azriel O, Bar-Haim Y. Attention bias. In: Abramowitz JS, editor. *Clinical Handbook of Fear and Anxiety: Maintenance Processes and Treatment Mechanisms.* American Psychological Association; 2020. pp. 203–18.

61 ***Interpretation bias refers*** Schoth and Liossi. A systematic review of experimental paradigms.

62 ***The task for those*** Beard, Cognitive bias modification for anxiety.

62   *The person doing* Schoth and Liossi, A systematic review of experimental paradigms for exploring biased interpretation.

62   *An exercise based on* Liu H, Li X, Han B, Liu X. Effects of cognitive bias modification on social anxiety: a meta-analysis. *PLoS One.* 2017 Apr 6;12(4):e0175107.

62   *An in-depth analysis* Fodor LA, Georgescu R, Cuijpers P, Szamoskozi Ş, David D, Furukawa TA, et al. Efficacy of cognitive bias modification interventions in anxiety and depressive disorders: a systematic review and network meta-analysis. *Lancet Psychiatry.* 2020 Jun;7(6):506–14.

64   *This creates the opportunity* Stubbs B, Vancampfort D, Rosenbaum S, Firth J, Cosco T, Veronese N, et al. An examination of the anxiolytic effects of exercise for people with anxiety and stress-related disorders: a meta-analysis. *J Psychiatry Res.* 2017 Mar;249: 102–8.

64   *In addition, research* Asmundson GJG, Fetzner MG, Deboer LB, Powers MB, Otto MW, Smits JAJ. Let's get physical: a contemporary review of the anxiolytic effects of exercise for anxiety and its disorders. *Depress Anxiety.* 2013 Apr;30(4):362–73.

64   *Thus, even doing something* Zelinger L, Zelinger J. *Please Explain Anxiety to Me!: Simple Biology and Solutions for Children and Parents.* Loving Healing Press; 2010.

64   *Along these lines* Croft A. Yoga as an intervention for anxiety in children and adolescents: a meta-analysis. Thesis. University of Adelaide. 2020. digital.library.adelaide.edu.au/dspace/handle /2440/131109

        Cramer H, Lauche R, Anheyer D, Pilkington K, de Manincor M, Dobos G, et al. Yoga for anxiety: a systematic review and meta-analysis of randomized controlled trials. *Depress Anxiety.* 2018 Sep;35(9):830–43.

64   *Yoga has also been* Chobe S, Chobe M, Metri K, Patra SK, Nagaratna R. Impact of yoga on cognition and mental health among elderly: a systematic review. *Complement Ther Med.* 2020 Aug;52: 102421.

64   *A closely related group* Kabat-Zinn J. *Mindfulness Meditation for Everyday Life.* Piatkus; 1994.

64 *Each moment lasts* Sauer S, Lemke J, Wittmann M, Kohls N, Mochty U, Walach H. How long is now for mindfulness meditators? *Pers Individ Dif.* 2012 Apr 1;52(6):750–4.

64 *Although most of* Drvaric L. Impact of one session of mindfulness vs. cognitive restructuring skills on worry and associated symptoms in generalized anxiety disorder. Thesis. McMaster University, Hamilton, Canada. 2013. macsphere.mcmaster.ca/bitstream/11375/13421/1/fulltext.pdf

65 *The growing demand* Oracle and Workplace Intelligence. AI@Work Global Research Report. 2020. oracle.com/a/ocom/docs/oracle-hcm-ai-at-work.pdf

65 *Even more astounding* Guo S, Deng W, Wang H, Liu J, Liu X, Yang X, et al. The efficacy of internet-based cognitive behavioural therapy for social anxiety disorder: a systematic review and meta-analysis. *Clin Psychol Psychother.* 2021 May;28(3):656–68.

Furmark T, Carlbring P, Hedman E, Sonnenstein A, Clevberger P, Bohman B, et al. Guided and unguided self-help for social anxiety disorder: randomised controlled trial. *Br J Psychiatry.* 2009 Nov;195(5):440–7.

Ivanova E, Lindner P, Ly KH, Dahlin M, Vernmark K, Andersson G, et al. Guided and unguided Acceptance and Commitment Therapy for social anxiety disorder and/or panic disorder provided via the internet and a smartphone application: a randomized controlled trial. *J Anxiety Disord.* 2016;44:27–35.

65 *Relaxation techniques as varied* Valmaggia LR, Latif L, Kempton MJ, Rus-Calafell M. Virtual reality in the psychological treatment for mental health problems: a systematic review of recent evidence. *Psychiatry Res.* 2016 Feb 28;236:189–95.

Pagnini F, Manzoni GM, Castelnuovo G, Molinari E. A brief literature review about relaxation therapy and anxiety. *Body Move Dance Psychother.* 2013 May 1;8(2):71–81.

66 *The positive impacts* Furmark et al., Guided and unguided self-help for social anxiety disorder.

Horigome T, Kurokawa S, Sawada K, Kudo S, Shiga K, Mimura M, et al. Virtual reality exposure therapy for social anxiety disorder: a systematic review and meta-analysis. *Psychol Med.* 2020 Nov;50(15):2487–97.

66 *This is illustrated* Zhang S, Chen M, Yang N, Lu S, Ni S. Effectiveness of VR based mindfulness on psychological and physiological health: a systematic review. *Curr Psychol.* 2021 May 19. link.springer.com/10.1007/s12144-021-01777-6

66 *This term was coined* Koerber B. What is the metaverse? A (kind of) simple explainer. Mashable. 2021 Nov 9. mashable.com/article/what-is-the-metaverse-explainer

66 *Your mind can also* Bem DJ. Self-perception theory. In: Berkowitz L, editor. *Advances in Experimental Social Psychology.* Academic Press; 1972. pp. 1–62.

   Dico GL. Self-perception theory, radical behaviourism, and the publicity/privacy issue. *Rev Philos Psychol.* 2018 Jun;9(2): 429–45.

67 *Taken together, all of this* Wilson TD. We are what we do. Edge.org. 2012. edge.org/response-detail/10281

67 *In 1979, a group* Langer EJ. *Counterclockwise: Mindful Health and the Power of Possibility.* Ballantine Books; 2009.

68 *This means having* Avvenuti G, Baiardini I, Giardini A. Optimism's explicative role for chronic diseases. *Front Psychol.* 2016 Mar 2;7:295.

68 *To get their baseline* Scheier MF, Carver CS, Bridges MW. Distinguishing optimism from neuroticism (and trait anxiety, self-mastery, and self-esteem): a reevaluation of the Life Orientation Test. *J Pers Soc Psychol.* 1994 Dec;67(6):1063–78.

69 *They found that each unit* Kim ES, Park N, Peterson C. Dispositional optimism protects older adults from stroke: the health and retirement study. *Stroke.* 2011 Oct;42(10):2855–9.

69 *Similarly, patients with* Novotny P, Colligan RC, Szydlo DW, Clark MM, Rausch S, Wampfler J, et al. A pessimistic explanatory style is prognostic for poor lung cancer survival. *J Thorac Oncol.* 2010 Mar 1;5(3):326–32.

69 *Optimism is also associated* Craig H, Freak-Poli R, Phyo AZZ, Ryan J, Gasevic D. The association of optimism and pessimism and all-cause mortality: a systematic review. *Pers Individ Dif.* 2021 Jul 1;177:110788.

69　*Another approach to self-creation* Wiggins JB. *Religion as Story.* Harper Forum Books. Harper and Row; 1975.

69　*According to this perspective* Randall WL. *The Stories We Are: An Essay on Self-Creation.* 2nd ed. University of Toronto Press; 2014.

69　*To do this successfully* Storr W. *The Science of Storytelling: Why Stories Make Us Human and How to Tell Them Better.* Abrams; 2020.

69　*In this way, you can direct* Creighton JL. Reframing your life story. *Psychol Today.* 2019 Sep 22. psychologytoday.com/ca/ blog/loving-through-your-differences/201909/reframing-your -life-story

70　*There is hardly* Kirsch I. Response expectancy as a determinant of experience and behavior. *Am Psychol.* 1985 Nov;40(11):1189– 202.

　　Colloca L, Miller FG. Role of expectations in health. *Curr Opin Psychiatry.* 2011 Mar;24(2):149–55.

70　*They found that* Wartolowska K, Judge A, Hopewell S, Collins GS, Dean BJF, Rombach I, et al. Use of placebo controls in the evaluation of surgery: systematic review. *BMJ.* 2014 May 21;348:g3253.

70　*The power of placebos* Kaptchuk TJ, Friedlander E, Kelley JM, Sanchez MN, Kokkotou E, Singer JP, et al. Placebos without deception: a randomized controlled trial in irritable bowel syndrome. *PLoS One.* 2010 Dec 22;5(12):e15591.

CHAPTER 6: SPACES MATTER

74　*Although the ideal amount* Leibold N. The effects of forest bathing on anxiety in adults: an integrative review. Paper. Department of Nursing, Southwest Minnesota State University. 2021. sigma .nursingrepository.org/handle/10755/21955

74　*Although more limited in size* Antonelli M, Donelli D, Carlone L, Maggini V, Firenzuoli F, Bedeschi E. Effects of forest bathing (shinrin-yoku) on individual well-being: an umbrella review. *Int J Environ Health Res.* 2021 Apr 28;1–26.

74 *Forest bathing seems* Wen Y, Yan Q, Pan Y, Gu X, Liu Y. Medical empirical research on forest bathing (shinrin-yoku): a systematic review. *Environ Health Prev Med.* 2019 Dec 1;24(1):70.

Bratman GN, Anderson CB, Berman MG, Cochran B, de Vries S, Flanders J, et al. Nature and mental health: an ecosystem service perspective. *Sci Adv.* 2019 Jul;5(7):eaax0903.

74 *People who live close* Carter M, Horwitz P. Beyond proximity: the importance of green space useability to self-reported health. *Ecohealth.* 2014 Sep;11(3):322–32.

White MP, Alcock I, Grellier J, Wheeler BW, Hartig T, Warber SL, et al. Spending at least 120 minutes a week in nature is associated with good health and wellbeing. *Sci Rep.* 2019 Jun 13;9(1):7730.

74 *Astoundingly, Green Spaces* Twohig-Bennett C, Jones A. The health benefits of the great outdoors: a systematic review and meta-analysis of greenspace exposure and health outcomes. *Environ Res.* 2018 Oct;166:628–37.

Gascon M, Triguero-Mas M, Martínez D, Dadvand P, Rojas-Rueda D, Plasència A, et al. Residential green spaces and mortality: a systematic review. *Environ Int.* 2016 Jan;86:60–7.

74 *A long-term project* Maes MJA, Pirani M, Booth ER, Shen C, Milligan B, Jones KE, et al. Benefit of woodland and other natural environments for adolescents' cognition and mental health. *Nat Sustain.* 2021 Jul 19;1–8.

75 *The potential large-scale* Robinson J, Breed M. Green prescriptions and their co-benefits: integrative strategies for public and environmental health. *Challenges.* 2019 Jan 17;10(1):9.

75 *you must be close enough* Wheeler BW, Lovell R, Higgins SL, White MP, Alcock I, Osborne NJ, et al. Beyond greenspace: an ecological study of population general health and indicators of natural environment type and quality. *Int J Health Geogr.* 2015 Apr 30;14:17.

Hermanski A, McClelland J, Pearce-Walker J, Ruiz J, Verhougstraete M. The effects of blue spaces on mental health and associated biomarkers. *Int J Ment Health.* 2021 Apr 20;1–15.

75 **Although Blue Spaces receive** Gascon M, Zijlema W, Vert C, White MP, Nieuwenhuijsen MJ. Outdoor blue spaces, human health and well-being: a systematic review of quantitative studies. *Int J Hyg Environ Health.* 2017 Nov;220(8):1207–21.

75 **People living near** Wheeler et al., Beyond greenspace.

Wheeler BW, White M, Stahl-Timmins W, Depledge MH. Does living by the coast improve health and wellbeing? *Health Place.* 2012 Sep;18(5):1198–201.

Finlay J, Franke T, McKay H, Sims-Gould J. Therapeutic landscapes and wellbeing in later life: impacts of blue and green spaces for older adults. *Health Place.* 2015 Jul;34:97–106.

Nutsford D, Pearson AL, Kingham S, Reitsma F. Residential exposure to visible blue space (but not green space) associated with lower psychological distress in a capital city. *Health Place.* 2016 May;39:70–8.

De Vries S, Ten Have M, van Dorsselaer S, van Wezep M, Hermans T, de Graaf R. Local availability of green and blue space and prevalence of common mental disorders in the Netherlands. *BJPsych Open.* 2016 Nov;2(6):366–72.

White MP, Alcock I, Wheeler BW, Depledge MH. Coastal proximity, health and well-being: results from a longitudinal panel survey. *Health Place.* 2013 Sep;23:97–103.

75 **They experience fewer** Völker S, Kistemann T. "I'm always entirely happy when I'm here!" Urban blue enhancing human health and well-being in Cologne and Düsseldorf, Germany. *Soc Sci Med.* 2013 Feb;78:113–24.

Grellier J, White MP, Albin M, Bell S, Elliott LR, Gascón M, et al. BlueHealth: a study programme protocol for mapping and quantifying the potential benefits to public health and well-being from Europe's blue spaces. *BMJ Open.* 2017 Jun 14;7(6):e016188.

75 **We respond positively** Miyazaki Y, Park B-J, Lee J. Nature therapy. In: Osaki M, Braimoh AK, Nakagami K, editors. *Designing Our Future: Local Perspectives on Bioproduction, Ecosystems and Humanity.* United Nations University Press; 2011. pp. 407–12.

Chang C-C, Cheng GJY, Nghiem TPL, Song XP, Oh RRY, Richards DR, et al. Social media, nature, and life satisfaction:

global evidence of the biophilia hypothesis. *Sci Rep.* 2020 Mar 5;10(1):4125.

76   ***Therefore, people tend*** Gifford R. Environmental psychology matters. *Annu Rev Psychol.* 2014;65:541–79.

76   ***Such restoration is facilitated*** Hartig T. Restoration in nature: beyond the conventional narrative. In: Schutte AR, Torquati JC, Stevens JR, editors. *Nature and Psychology: Biological, Cognitive, Developmental, and Social Pathways to Well-Being.* Springer International; 2021. pp. 89–151.

     Grinde B, Patil GG. Biophilia: does visual contact with nature impact on health and well-being? *Int J Environ Res Public Health.* 2009 Sep;6(9):2332–43.

76   ***In other words*** Ulrich RS, Simons RF, Losito BD, Fiorito E, Miles MA, Zelson M. Stress recovery during exposure to natural and urban environments. *J Environ Psychol.* 1991 Sep 1;11(3): 201–30.

76   ***Since most people*** Deng L, Deng Q. The basic roles of indoor plants in human health and comfort. *Environ Sci Pollut Res Int.* 2018 Dec;25(36):36087–101.

     Klepeis NE, Nelson WC, Ott WR, Robinson JP, Tsang AM, Switzer P, et al. The National Human Activity Pattern Survey (NHAPS): a resource for assessing exposure to environmental pollutants. *J Expo Sci Environ Epidemiol.* 2001 Jul 26;11(3): 231–52.

     Tarrat C. The indoor generation. Get Outdoors. 2018. getout doorsuk.org/blogs/news/the-indoor-generation

76   ***This is the group*** Buitrago Restrepo F, Duque Marquez I. *The Orange Economy: An Infinite Opportunity.* Inter-American Development Bank; 2013. publications.iadb.org/en/orange-economy -infinite-opportunity

77   ***Just visiting a museum*** Chatterjee H, Noble G. *Museums, Health and Well-Being.* 1st ed. Taylor and Francis; 2017.

     Dodd J, Jones C. Mind, body, spirit: how museums impact health and wellbeing. Report. Research Centre for Museums and Galleries, School of Museum Studies, University of Leices-

ter. 2014. southeastmuseums.org/wp-content/uploads/PDF/mind
_body_spirit_report.pdf

77   *Women visiting art exhibitions* Nummela O, Sulander T, Rah-
      konen O, Uutela A. Associations of self-rated health with differ-
      ent forms of leisure activities among ageing people. *Int J Public
      Health.* 2008;53(5):227–35.

77   *The same is true* Colenberg S, Jylhä T, Arkesteijn M. The relation-
      ship between interior office space and employee health and well-
      being—a literature review. *Build Res Inf.* 2021;49(3):352–66.

77   *Some scholars and designers* Ulrich RS. Effects of gardens on
      health outcomes: theory and research. In: Marcus CC, Barnes M,
      editors. *Healing Gardens: Therapeutic Benefits and Design Recom-
      mendations.* New York: Wiley; 1999. pp. 27–86.

78   *Architecture seems to have* Kraftl P, Adey P. Architecture/affect/
      inhabitation: geographies of being-in buildings. *Ann Assoc Am
      Geogr.* 2008 Feb 5;98(1):213–31.
          Rose G, Degen M, Basdas B. More on "big things": building
      events and feelings. *Trans Inst Br Geogr.* 2010 Apr 15;35(3):
      334–49.

78   *Somehow, the design briefs* Deppeler J, Aikens K. Responsible
      innovation in school design—a systematic review. *J Responsible
      Innov.* 2020 Sep 1;7(3):573–97.

78   *Physical constructions can* Evans GW. The built environment
      and mental health. *J Urban Health.* 2003 Dec;80(4):536–55.

79   *"Innovation" in this space goes* Kerr J, Carlson JA, Sallis JF,
      Rosenberg D, Leak CR, Saelens BE, et al. Assessing health-related
      resources in senior living residences. *J Aging Stud.* 2011
      Aug;25(3):206–14.

79   *They are designed* Fox NJ. Creativity and health: an anti-
      humanist reflection. *Health.* 2013 Sep;17(5):495–511.

80   *This setting would enable* Vinick D. Dementia-friendly design:
      Hogeweyk and beyond. *Br J Gen Pract.* 2019 Jun;69(683):300.

81   *As a result, the need* Godwin B. Hogewey: a "home from home" in
      the Netherlands. *J Dement Care.* 2015;23(3):28–31.

81 *After they moved to Hogewey* Harris J, Topfer LA, Ford C. Dementia villages: innovative residential care for people with dementia. *CADTH Issues in Emerging Health Technologies.* CADTH. 2019 Oct. cadth.ca/sites/default/files/hs-eh/eh0071 -dementia-villages.pdf

81 *As far back as 500 B.C.* Hippocrates. On Airs, Waters, and Places. Adams F, translator. The Internet Classics Archive. classics.mit .edu/Hippocrates/airwatpl.1.1.html
   Stichler JF. Healing by design. *J Nurs Adm.* 2008 Dec;38(12): 505–9.

82 *When the few medicines* Schweitzer M, Gilpin L, Frampton S. Healing spaces: elements of environmental design that make an impact on health. *J Altern Complement Med.* 2004 Oct 1;10(Suppl 1):S71–83.

82 *These types of surroundings* Lyons AS, Petrucelli JR. *Medicine: An Illustrated History.* 1st ed. Abrams; 1978.

82 *The word comes from* Had a long day of travel? Check into a hospital. Merriam-Webster. 2017. merriam-webster.com/words-at -play/word-history-hospital-hostel-hotel-hospice

82 *The shift in the sense* Hospital. Online Etymology Dictionary. Accessed 2022 Apr 27. etymonline.com/word/hospital

82 *As antibiotics were introduced* Serra M, Palacio DO, Espinal S, Rodriguez DG, Jadad AR. *Trusted Networks: The Key to Achieve World-Class Health Outcomes on a Shoestring.* Beati; 2018.

83 *Their designs became* Speciale ZS. Humanizing where we heal: an examination of healthcare aesthetics and evidence-based hospital design. Thesis. Baylor University. 2020. baylor-ir.tdl .org/bitstream/handle/2104/11165/Zachary_Speciale1 _honorsthesis.pdf?sequence=1

83 *Investigations into hospital design* Ulrich RS. Effects of interior design on wellness: theory and recent scientific research. *J Health Care Inter Des.* 1991;3:97–109.

83 *These realizations have* Gesler WM. Therapeutic landscapes: theory and a case study of Epidauros, Greece. *Environ Plan D.* 1993 Apr 1;11(2):171–89.

83   *Explorations in these spaces* Lea J. Retreating to nature: rethinking "therapeutic landscapes." *Area.* 2008 Mar;40(1):90–8.

83   *As this wave of innovation* Escobar YP. Cuidar de la salud y no solo de la enfermedad. Universidad de Antioquia. 2009.

84   *This initiative, the* North Hawaiʻi Community Hospital. EarlBakken.com. earlbakken.com/content/involvement/north .hawaii.community.hospital.html

85   *It combined top* Becker NB. Healing journey spans high-tech, high-touch at Hawaiian hospital. *Altern Ther Health Med.* 2000 Mar;6(2):99–100.

85   *Changes like simply adding* Park S-H, Mattson RH. Ornamental indoor plants in hospital rooms enhanced health outcomes of patients recovering from surgery. *J Altern Complement Med.* 2009 Sep;15(9):975–80.

85   *As this type of relationship* Jacobs JM. A geography of big things. *Cult Geogr.* 2006 Jan 1;13(1):1–27.

86   *You can reduce* Yeo LB. Psychological and physiological benefits of plants in the indoor environment: a mini and in-depth review. *Int J Built Environ Sustain.* 2021;8(1):57–67.

      Mo L, Ma Z, Xu Y, Sun F, Lun X, Liu X, et al. Assessing the capacity of plant species to accumulate particulate matter in Beijing, China. *PLoS One.* 2015 Oct 27;10(10):e0140664.

86   *Offices with plants* Bergefurt L, Weijs-Perrée M, Appel-Meulenbroek R, Arentze T. The physical office workplace as a resource for mental health—a systematic scoping review. *Build Environ.* 2022 Jan 1;207:108505.

86   *Whatever type of* Soga M, Gaston KJ, Yamaura Y. Gardening is beneficial for health: a meta-analysis. *Prev Med Rep.* 2017 Mar 1;5:92–9.

CHAPTER 7: TRUST YOUR GUT

87   *In the year 2000* Berdoy M, Webster JP, Macdonald DW. Fatal attraction in rats infected with Toxoplasma gondii. *Proc Biol Sci.* 2000 Aug 7;267(1452):1591–4.

87 *The benefit to the toxo* Mendonça-Natividade FC, Ricci-Azevedo R. Toxoplasma gondii: a microbe that turns mice into zombies. *Front Young Minds.* 2020 Mar 31;8. frontiersin.org/article/10.3389/frym.2020.00036/full

87 *Since the 1950s* Buentello E. Preliminary observations on the relationship between toxoplasmosis, lysergic acid and schizophrenia [in Spanish]. *Gac Med Mex.* 1958;88(10):693–708.

87 *International evidence indicates* Underwood E. Reality check: can cat poop cause mental illness? *Science.* 2019. sciencemag.org/news/2019/02/reality-check-can-cat-poop-cause-mental-illness

Molan A, Nosaka K, Hunter M, Wang W. Global status of Toxoplasma gondii infection: systematic review and prevalence snapshots. *Trop Biomed.* 2019 Dec 1;36(4):898–925.

87 *It has been found, for example* Lerner DA, Alkaersig L, Fitza MA, Lomberg C, Johnson SK. Nothing ventured, nothing gained: parasite infection is associated with entrepreneurial initiation, engagement, and performance. *Entrep Theory Pract.* 2021 Jan 1;45(1):118–44.

Plackett B. Can a cat parasite control your mind? Life's little mysteries. Live Science. 2020 Oct 3. livescience.com/can-cat-parasites-control-human-brains.html

88 *Of those, 14 percent* Johnson SK, Fitza MA, Lerner DA, Calhoun DM, Beldon MA, Chan ET, et al. Risky business: linking Toxoplasma gondii infection and entrepreneurship behaviours across individuals and countries. *Proc Biol Sci.* 2018 Jul 25; 285(1883). dx.doi.org/10.1098/rspb.2018.0822

88 *Similarly, a study in Denmark* Lerner et al., Nothing ventured, nothing gained.

88 *It may also reflect* Martinez VO, de Mendonça Lima FW, de Carvalho CF, Menezes-Filho JA. Toxoplasma gondii infection and behavioral outcomes in humans: a systematic review. *Parasitol Res.* 2018 Oct;117(10):3059–65.

Lerner et al., Nothing ventured, nothing gained.

89 *People with positive tests* Peng X, Brenner LA, Mathai AJ, Cook TB, Fuchs D, Postolache N, et al. Moderation of the relationship between Toxoplasma gondii seropositivity and trait im-

pulsivity in younger men by the phenylalanine-tyrosine ratio. *Psychiatry Res.* 2018 Dec;270:992–1000.

89   *The conditions that toxo seems* Nayeri Chegeni T, Sarvi S, Amouei A, Moosazadeh M, Hosseininejad Z, Aghayan SA, et al. Relationship between toxoplasmosis and obsessive compulsive disorder: a systematic review and meta-analysis. *PLoS Negl Trop Dis.* 2019 Apr;13(4):e0007306.

      Bayani M, Riahi SM, Bazrafshan N, Ray Gamble H, Rostami A. Toxoplasma gondii infection and risk of Parkinson and Alzheimer diseases: a systematic review and meta-analysis on observational studies. *Acta Trop.* 2019 Aug;196:165–71.

      Flegr J, Horáček J. Negative effects of latent toxoplasmosis on mental health. *Front Psychiatry.* 2019;10:1012.

89   *above all, schizophrenia* Smith G. Estimating the population attributable fraction for schizophrenia when Toxoplasma gondii is assumed absent in human populations. *Prev Vet Med.* 2014 Dec 1;117(3–4):425–35.

89   *On top of that* Samojłowicz D, Borowska-Solonynko A, Kruczyk M. New, previously unreported correlations between latent Toxoplasma gondii infection and excessive ethanol consumption. *Forensic Sci Int.* 2017 Nov;280:49–54.

      Amouei A, Moosazadeh M, Nayeri Chegeni T, Sarvi S, Mizani A, Pourasghar M, et al. Evolutionary puzzle of Toxoplasma gondii with suicidal ideation and suicide attempts: an updated systematic review and meta-analysis. *Transbound Emerg Dis.* 2020 Mar 21. onlinelibrary.wiley.com/doi/10.1111/tbed.13550

89   *It has been estimated* Milne G, Webster JP, Walker M. Toxoplasma gondii: an underestimated threat? *Trends Parasitol.* 2020 Dec;36(12):959–69.

90   *By this measure alone* Sender R, Fuchs S, Milo R. Revised estimates for the number of human and bacteria cells in the body. *PLoS Biol.* 2016 Aug;14(8):e1002533.

90   *It is currently estimated* Willyard C. New human gene tally reignites debate. *Nature.* 2018 Jun;558(7710):354–5.

90   *2 million to 20 million* Knight R, Callewaert C, Marotz C, Hyde ER, Debelius JW, McDonald D, et al. The microbiome and

human biology. *Annu Rev Genomics Hum Genet.* 2017 Aug 31;18:65–86.

90   *According to that estimate* Nicholson A, Negussie Y, Shah CM, Ayano Ogawa V. Microbial dimension to human development and well-being. In: National Academies of Sciences, Engineering, and Medicine. *The Convergence of Infectious Diseases and Non-communicable Diseases: Proceedings of a Workshop.* National Academies Press; 2019. pp. 51–63.

  Turnbaugh PJ, Ley RE, Hamady M, Fraser-Liggett CM, Knight R, Gordon JI. The human microbiome project. *Nature.* 2007 Oct 18;449(7164):804–10.

90   *Those in your mouth* Deo PN, Deshmukh R. Oral microbiome: unveiling the fundamentals. *J Oral Maxillofac Pathol.* 2019 Jan;23(1):122–8.

90   *Those in your gut* Ferranti EP, Dunbar SB, Dunlop AL, Corwin EJ. 20 things you didn't know about the human gut microbiome. *J Cardiovasc Nurs.* 2014 Nov;29(6):479–81.

91   *Your skin's microbiome* Eisenstein M. The skin microbiome. *Nature.* 2020 Dec;588(7838):s209.

91   *The microorganisms found* Rowe M, Veerus L, Trosvik P, Buckling A, Pizzari T. The reproductive microbiome: an emerging driver of sexual selection, sexual conflict, mating systems, and reproductive isolation. *Trends Ecol Evol.* 2020 Mar;35(3):220–34.

91   *Those in your lungs* Mathieu E, Escribano-Vazquez U, Descamps D, Cherbuy C, Langella P, Riffault S, et al. Paradigms of lung microbiota functions in health and disease, particularly, in asthma. *Front Physiol.* 2018 Aug 21;9:1168.

91   *The recognition that most* Margulis L. *Symbiotic Planet: A New Look at Evolution.* Basic Books; 2008.

91   *Instead of an organism* Gilbert SF, Sapp J, Tauber AI. A symbiotic view of life: we have never been individuals. *Q Rev Biol.* 2012 Dec;87(4):325–41.

  Salvucci E. Microbiome, holobiont and the net of life. *Crit Rev Microbiol.* 2016 May;42(3):485–94.

  Van de Guchte M, Blottière HM, Doré J. Humans as holobionts: implications for prevention and therapy. *Microbiome.* 2018 Dec;6(1). dx.doi.org/10.1186/s40168-018-0466-8

91 *After all, an organ* Neumann PE. Organ or not? Prolegomenon to organology. *Clin Anat.* 2017 Apr;30(3):288–9.

92 *This applies to the gut* Patra V, Wagner K, Arulampalam V, Wolf P. Skin microbiome modulates the effect of ultraviolet radiation on cellular response and immune function. *iScience.* 2019 May 31;15:211–22.

92 *Furthermore, the microbial communities* Coscia A, Bardanzellu F, Caboni E, Fanos V, Peroni DG. When a neonate is born, so is a microbiota. *Life (Basel).* 2021 Feb 16;11(2):148.

Looi M-K. The human microbiome: everything you need to know about the 39 trillion microbes that call our bodies home. *BBC Science Focus Magazine.* 2020 Jul 14. sciencefocus.com/the -human-body/human-microbiome

92 *This dialogue between* Berding K, Vlckova K, Marx W, Schellekens H, Stanton C, Clarke G, et al. Diet and the microbiota-gut-brain axis: sowing the seeds of good mental health. *Adv Nutr.* 2021;12(4):1–47. doi.org/10.1093/advances/nmaa181

92 *Another is the liver* Albillos A, de Gottardi A, Rescigno M. The gut-liver axis in liver disease: pathophysiological basis for therapy. *J Hepatol.* 2020 Mar;72(3):558–77.

92 *Interestingly, imbalances* Stavropoulou E, Kantartzi K, Tsigalou C, Konstantinidis T, Romanidou G, Voidarou C, et al. Focus on the gut-kidney axis in health and disease. *Front Med.* 2020; 7:620102.

Yang T, Richards EM, Pepine CJ, Raizada MK. The gut microbiota and the brain-gut-kidney axis in hypertension and chronic kidney disease. *Nat Rev Nephrol.* 2018 Jul;14(7):442–56.

93 *Lastly, perhaps the richest* Enaud R, Prevel R, Ciarlo E, Beaufils F, Wieërs G, Guery B, et al. The gut-lung axis in health and respiratory diseases: a place for inter-organ and inter-kingdom crosstalks. *Front Cell Infect Microbiol.* 2020 Feb 19;10:9.

93 *The connections between* Kim YJ, Womble JT, Gunsch CK, Ingram JL. The gut/lung microbiome axis in obesity, asthma, and

bariatric surgery: a literature review. *Obesity*. 2021 Apr;29(4): 636–44.

93   ***Low microbiome diversity*** Hugerth LW, Andreasson A, Talley NJ, Forsberg AM, Kjellström L, Schmidt PT, et al. No distinct microbiome signature of irritable bowel syndrome found in a Swedish random population. *Gut*. 2020 Jun;69(6):1076–84.

93   ***This is the result of less*** Jandhyala SM, Talukdar R, Subramanyam C, Vuyyuru H, Sasikala M, Nageshwar Reddy D. Role of the normal gut microbiota. *World J Gastroenterol*. 2015 Aug 7; 21(29):8787–803.

      DeGruttola AK, Low D, Mizoguchi A, Mizoguchi E. Current understanding of dysbiosis in disease in human and animal models. *Inflamm Bowel Dis*. 2016 May;22(5):1137–50.

93   ***A westernized diet*** Koszewicz M, Jaroch J, Brzecka A, Ejma M, Budrewicz S, Mikhaleva LM, et al. Dysbiosis is one of the risk factors for stroke and cognitive impairment and potential target for treatment. *Pharmacol Res*. 2021 Feb;164:105277.

      Sublette ME, Cheung S, Lieberman E, Hu S, Mann JJ, Uhlemann A-C, et al. Bipolar disorder and the gut microbiome: a systematic review. *Bipolar Disord*. 2021 Jan 29. dx.doi.org/10.1111/bdi.13049

      Verma H, Phian S, Lakra P, Kaur J, Subudhi S, Lal R, et al. Human gut microbiota and mental health: advancements and challenges in microbe-based therapeutic interventions. *Indian J Microbiol*. 2020 Dec;60(4):405–19.

94   ***These problems are*** Kopp W. How Western diet and lifestyle drive the pandemic of obesity and civilization diseases. *Diabetes Metab Syndr Obes*. 2019 Oct 24;12:2221–36.

94   ***The recognition of*** Mohanty S, Singhal K. Functional foods as personalised nutrition: definitions and genomic insights. In: Rani V, Yadav UCS, editors. *Functional Food and Human Health*. Springer Singapore; 2018. pp. 513–35.

94   ***The purpose of*** Tufarelli V, Laudadio V. An overview on the functional food concept: prospectives and applied researches in probiotics, prebiotics and synbiotics. *J Exp Biol Agric Sci*. 2016 May 25;4(3)(Suppl):273–8.

Braconi D, Bernardini G, Millucci L, Santucci A. Foodomics for human health: current status and perspectives. *Expert Rev Proteomics.* 2018 Feb;15(2):153–64.

Salminen S, Collado MC, Endo A, Hill C, Lebeer S, Quigley EMM, et al. The International Scientific Association of Probiotics and Prebiotics (ISAPP) consensus statement on the definition and scope of postbiotics. *Nat Rev Gastroenterol Hepatol.* 2021 May 4. dx.doi.org/10.1038/s41575-021-00440-6

Smith LK, Wissel EF. Microbes and the mind: how bacteria shape affect, neurological processes, cognition, social relationships, development, and pathology. *Perspect Psychol Sci.* 2019 May;14(3):397–418.

95 **It has been used** De Groot PF, Frissen MN, de Clercq NC, Nieuwdorp M. Fecal microbiota transplantation in metabolic syndrome: history, present and future. *Gut Microbes.* 2017 May 4;8(3):253–67.

95 **Curiously, many animals** Lewin RA. *Merde: Excursions in Scientific, Cultural, and Socio-historical Coprology.* Random House; 2009.

95 **The scientific foundations** Dobell C. The discovery of the intestinal protozoa of man. *Proc R Soc Med.* 1920 Nov 1;13(Sect Hist Med):1–15.

95 **the first medical book** Monestier M. *Histoire et bizarreries sociales des excréments: des origines à nos jours.* Cherche midi; 1997.

95 **After the extensive characterization** Lewin, *Merde.*

95 **This bacterium can** Scott RD II, Slayton RB, Lessa FC, Baggs J, Culler SD, McDonald LC, et al. Assessing the social cost and benefits of a national requirement establishing antibiotic stewardship programs to prevent Clostridioides difficile infection in US hospitals. *Antimicrob Resist Infect Control.* 2019 Jan 22;8:17.

95 **Clinical trials studying** Baunwall SMD, Lee MM, Eriksen MK, Mullish BH, Marchesi JR, Dahlerup JF, et al. Faecal microbiota transplantation for recurrent Clostridioides difficile infection: an updated systematic review and meta-analysis. *EClinicalMedicine.* 2020 Dec;29–30:100642.

96   *Studies showed that* De Groot P, Nikolic T, Pellegrini S, Sordi V, Imangaliyev S, Rampanelli E, et al. Faecal microbiota transplantation halts progression of human new-onset type 1 diabetes in a randomised controlled trial. *Gut.* 2021 Jan;70(1):92–105.

       Baruch EN, Youngster I, Ben-Betzalel G, Ortenberg R, Lahat A, Katz L, et al. Fecal microbiota transplant promotes response in immunotherapy-refractory melanoma patients. *Science.* 2021 Feb 5;371(6529):602–9.

96   *Other studies went* Chinna Meyyappan A, Forth E, Wallace CJK, Milev R. Effect of fecal microbiota transplant on symptoms of psychiatric disorders: a systematic review. *BMC Psychiatry.* 2020 Jun 15;20(1):299.

97   *In addition to revealing* Milo R, Phillips R. How quickly do different cells in the body replace themselves? In: *Cell Biology by the Numbers.* Garland Science; 2015. book.bionumbers.org/how-quickly-do-different-cells-in-the-body-replace-themselves

98   *By feeling strongly* Struhl KJ. What kind of an illusion is the illusion of self. *Comp Philos.* 2020;11(2):8.

98   *These stories then* Mead GH. *Mind, Self, and Society: The Definitive Edition.* University of Chicago Press; 2015.

       Hood B. *The Self Illusion: How the Social Brain Creates Identity.* Oxford University Press; 2012.

98   *The experience of* Oliver T. *The Self Delusion: The Surprising Science of Our Connection to Each Other and the Natural World.* Hachette UK; 2020.

       Metzinger T. *The Ego Tunnel: The Science of the Mind and the Myth of the Self.* Basic Books; 2009.

CHAPTER 8: THE COMPANY YOU KEEP

100   *The brain hemorrhage* Bruenn HG. Clinical notes on the illness and death of President Franklin D. Roosevelt. *Ann Intern Med.* 1970 Apr 1;72(4):579–91.

100   *There was such a poor* Mahmood SS, Levy D, Vasan RS, Wang TJ. The Framingham Heart Study and the epidemiology of

cardiovascular disease: a historical perspective. *Lancet.* 2014 Mar 15;383(9921):999–1008.

101 *As a result, it was* Research milestones. Framingham Heart Study. 2017. web.archive.org/web/20170710153926/http://www.framinghamheartstudy.org/about-fhs/research-milestones.php

101 *Such insights led to* Tsao CW, Vasan RS. The Framingham Heart Study: past, present and future. *Int J Epidemiol.* 2015 Dec;44(6): 1763–6.

102 *Furthermore, when any two* Christakis NA, Fowler JH. The spread of obesity in a large social network over 32 years. *N Engl J Med.* 2007 Jul 26;357(4):370–9.

102 *In general, a human network* Mata AS da. Complex networks: a mini-review. *Braz J Phys.* 2020 Oct 1;50(5):658–72.

102 *Your social network* Chami GF, Ahnert SE, Voors MJ, Kontoleon AA. Social network analysis predicts health behaviours and self-reported health in African villages. *PLoS One.* 2014 Jul 29;9(7):e103500.
    Kingsford RL. Self-rated health and community/social relations. Thesis. Utah State University. 2008. digitalcommons.usu.edu/etd/98

103 *they can contribute financially* Berkman LF, Glass T, Brissette I, Seeman TE. From social integration to health: Durkheim in the new millennium. *Soc Sci Med.* 2000 Sep;51(6):843–57.

103 *People with large* Windsor TD, Rioseco P, Fiori KL, Curtis RG, Booth H. Structural and functional social network attributes moderate the association of self-rated health with mental health in midlife and older adults. *Int Psychogeriatr.* 2016 Jan;28(1): 49–61.

103 *The health effects of* Jia H, Lubetkin EI. Life expectancy and active life expectancy by marital status among older U.S. adults: results from the U.S. Medicare Health Outcome Survey (HOS). *SSM Popul Health.* 2020 Dec 1;12:100642.

103 *These people experience* Adelman RD, Tmanova LL, Delgado D, Dion S, Lachs MS. Caregiver burden: a clinical review. *JAMA.* 2014 Mar 12;311(10):1052–60.

Del-Pino-Casado R, Priego-Cubero E, López-Martínez C, Orgeta V. Subjective caregiver burden and anxiety in informal caregivers: a systematic review and meta-analysis. *PLoS One.* 2021 Mar 1;16(3):e0247143.

Schiller VF, Dorstyn DS, Taylor AM. The protective role of social support sources and types against depression in caregivers: a meta-analysis. *J Autism Dev Disord.* 2021 Apr;51(4):1304–15.

Rico-Uribe LA, Caballero FF, Martín-María N, Cabello M, Ayuso-Mateos JL, Miret M. Association of loneliness with all-cause mortality: a meta-analysis. *PLoS One.* 2018 Jan 4;13(1): e0190033.

103 *Your likelihood of having* Montgomery SC, Donnelly M, Bhatnagar P, Carlin A, Kee F, Hunter RF. Peer social network processes and adolescent health behaviors: a systematic review. *Prev Med.* 2020 Jan;130:105900.

Henneberger AK, Mushonga DR, Preston AM. Peer influence and adolescent substance use: a systematic review of dynamic social network research. *Adolesc Res Rev.* 2021 Mar;6(1):57–73.

Leonardi-Bee J, Jere ML, Britton J. Exposure to parental and sibling smoking and the risk of smoking uptake in childhood and adolescence: a systematic review and meta-analysis. *Thorax.* 2011 Oct;66(10):847–55.

103 *The effects of these* Blumer H. Collective behavior. In: Park RE, editor. *An Outline of the Principles of Sociology.* Barnes and Noble; 1939. pp. 219–80.

Levy DA, Nail PR. Contagion: a theoretical and empirical review and reconceptualization. *Genet Soc Gen Psychol Monogr.* 1993 May;119(2):233–84.

104 *News stories about* Wood S, Bollinger B. Predicting changes in patient choice of preventive health care after celebrity diagnoses. *JACR.* 2020 Jul 1;5(3):302–10.

104 *The same thing can occur* Domaradzki J. The Werther effect, the Papageno effect or no effect? A literature review. *Int J Environ Res Public Health.* 2021 Mar 1;18(5): 2396.

104 *Social contagion can also* Christakis NA, Fowler JH. Social contagion theory: examining dynamic social networks and human behavior. *Stat Med.* 2013 Feb 20;32(4):556–77.

Fowler JH, Christakis NA. Dynamic spread of happiness in a large social network: longitudinal analysis over 20 years in the Framingham Heart Study. *BMJ.* 2008 Dec 4;337:a2338.

Christakis NA, Fowler JH. The collective dynamics of smoking in a large social network. *N Engl J Med.* 2008 May 22;358(21): 2249–58.

104 ***Companies, another network*** Kensbock JM, Alkaersig L, Lomberg C. The epidemic of mental disorders in business— how depression, anxiety, and stress spread across organizations through employee mobility. *Adm Sci Q.* 2021 May 18; 00018392211014819.

105 ***Friendship is so powerful*** Dunbar RIM. The anatomy of friendship. *Trends Cogn Sci.* 2018 Jan;22(1):32–51.

105 ***Men without friends*** Almquist YM. Childhood friendships and adult health: findings from the Aberdeen Children of the 1950s cohort study. *Eur J Public Health.* 2012 Jun;22(3):378–83.

105 ***In contrast, having close*** Ho CY. Better health with more friends: the role of social capital in producing health. *Health Econ.* 2016 Jan;25(1):91–100.

Waxler-Morrison N, Hislop TG, Mears B, Kan L. Effects of social relationships on survival for women with breast cancer: a prospective study. *Soc Sci Med.* 1991;33(2):177–83.

Dunbar, The anatomy of friendship.

Holt-Lunstad J, Smith TB, Layton JB. Social relationships and mortality risk: a meta-analytic review. *PLoS Med.* 2010 Jul 27;7(7):e1000316.

106 ***Ordinarily, each person*** Mac Carron P, Kaski K, Dunbar R. Calling Dunbar's numbers. *Soc Networks.* 2016 Oct 1;47:151–5.

106 ***The word "friend"*** Amichai-Hamburger Y, Kingsbury M, Schneider BH. Friendship: an old concept with a new meaning? *Comput Human Behav.* 2013 Jan 1;29(1):33–9.

Vernon M. *The Meaning of Friendship.* Springer; 2016.

Hojjat M, Moyer A, Halpin AM. *The Psychology of Friendship.* Oxford University Press; 2017.

106 ***One of the main barriers*** Andersson L. Loneliness research and interventions: a review of the literature. *Aging Ment Health.* 1998 Nov 1;2(4):264–74.

Rook KS. Research on social support, loneliness, and social isolation: toward an integration. *Pers Soc Psychol Rev.* 1984;5: 239–64.

107 ***Based on data collected*** Hammond C. The surprising truth about loneliness. *BBC Future.* 2018 Sep 30. bbc.com/future/article /20180928-the-surprising-truth-about-loneliness

Barreto M, Victor C, Hammond C, Eccles A, Richins MT, Qualter P. Loneliness around the world: age, gender, and cultural differences in loneliness. *Pers Individ Dif.* 2021 Feb 1;169:110066.

107 ***The numbers in the US*** Loneliness and the workplace. Cigna. 2020. cigna.com/static/www-cigna-com/docs/about-us/newsroom /studies-and-reports/combatting-loneliness/cigna-2020-loneli ness-factsheet.pdf

107 ***The prevalence of loneliness*** Hajek A, Kretzler B, König H-H. Multimorbidity, loneliness, and social isolation. a systematic review. *Int J Environ Res Public Health.* 2020 Nov 23;17(22). dx.doi.org/10.3390/ijerph17228688

107 ***In fact, analysis of data*** Holt-Lunstad J, Smith TB, Baker M, Harris T, Stephenson D. Loneliness and social isolation as risk factors for mortality: a meta-analytic review. *Perspect Psychol Sci.* 2015 Mar;10(2):227–37.

The "Loneliness Epidemic." Health Resources and Services Administration. 2019 Jan. hrsa.gov/enews/past-issues/2019/ january-17/loneliness-epidemic

107 ***What adds to the concern*** Cacioppo JT, Cacioppo S. The growing problem of loneliness. *Lancet.* 2018 Feb 3;391(10119):426.

107 ***Even though many interventions*** National Academies of Sciences, Engineering, and Medicine. *Social Isolation and Loneliness in Older Adults: Opportunities for the Health Care System.* National Academies Press; 2020.

108 ***These interventions tend*** Gasteiger N, Loveys K, Law M, Broadbent E. Friends from the future: a scoping review of research into robots and computer agents to combat loneliness in older people. *Clin Interv Aging.* 2021 May 24;16:941–71.

109 *As the name indicates* Hernandez D. What is an affinity group? Resilience Circles. 2012 May 17. localcircles.org/2012/05/17/ what-is-an-affinity-group

109 *the protests against* Peeples JA, Mitchell B. "No mobs—no confusions—no tumult": networking civil disobedience. *J Commun.* 2007;17(1–2). cios.org/EJCPUBLIC/017/1/01714.html

109 *Extinction Rebellion* Why rebel. Extinction Rebellion. rebellion .global/why-rebel

109 *Perhaps the most* Ahern S, Bailey KG. *Family-by-Choice: Creating Family in a World of Strangers.* Fairview Press; 1996.

109 *For a proactive social network* Serra M, Palacio DO, Espinal S, Rodriguez DG, Jadad AR. *Trusted Networks: The Key to Achieve World-Class Health Outcomes on a Shoestring.* Beati; 2018.

110 *It is said that* Stevens DP. Handovers and Debussy. *Qual Saf Health Care.* 2008 Feb;17(1):2–3.

110 *The word "connection"* Connect. Online Etymology Dictionary. Accessed 2022 Apr 27. etymonline.com/search?q=connect

112 *To raise the stakes even further* Secretary-general calls latest IPCC climate report "code red for humanity," stressing "irrefutable" evidence of human influence. Report. United Nations. 2021 Aug 9. un.org/press/en/2021/sgsm20847.doc.htm

Climate change 2021: the physical science basis. Intergovernmental Panel on Climate Change. 2021. ipcc.ch/report/sixth -assessment-report-working-group-i

Rocque RJ, Beaudoin C, Ndjaboue R, Cameron L, Poirier-Bergeron L, Poulin-Rheault R-A, et al. Health effects of climate change: an overview of systematic reviews. *BMJ Open.* 2021 Jun 9;11(6):e046333.

112 *That was 3 times* Landrigan PJ, Fuller R, Acosta NJR, Adeyi O, Arnold R, Basu NN, et al. The Lancet Commission on pollution and health. *Lancet.* 2018 Feb 3;391(10119):462–512.

112 *Furthermore, more than 70 percent* Fuller R, Rahona E, Fisher S, Caravanos J, Webb D, Kass D, et al. Pollution and non-communicable disease: time to end the neglect. *Lancet Planet Health.* 2018 Mar;2(3):e96–8.

CHAPTER 9: GETTING OUT OF YOUR OWN WAY

113 *The thick-footed morel* Sheldrake M. *Entangled Life: How Fungi Make Our Worlds, Change Our Minds and Shape Our Futures.* Random House; 2020.

113 *In addition, we are not* Hogenboom M. Humans are nowhere near as special as we like to think. *BBC Earth.* 2015 Jul 3.

114 *This evidence has motivated* Gordon J-S. Artificial moral and legal personhood. *AI Soc.* 2021 Jun;36(2):457–71.

114 *Even our darkest qualities* Palmer CT. Rape in nonhuman animal species: definitions, evidence, and implications. *J Sex Res.* 1989;26(3):355–74.

Castro J. Do animals murder each other? *Live Science.* 2017 Sep 16. livescience.com/60431-do-animals-murder-each-other .html

114 *We have already created* Wilson M. AI is inventing languages humans can't understand. Should we stop it? *Fast Company.* 2017 Jul 14. fastcompany.com/90132632/ai-is-inventing-its-own-perfect -languages-should-we-let-it

114 *learning to cooperate* Crandall JW, Oudah M, Tennom, Ishowo-Oloko F, Abdallah S, Bonnefon J-F, et al. Cooperating with machines. *Nat Commun.* 2018 Jan 16;9(1):233.

114 *even ask questions* Yuan X, Wang T, Gulcehre C, Sordoni A, Bachman P, Subramanian S, et al. Machine comprehension by text-to-text neural question generation. *arXiv.* 2017 May; 1705.02012 [cs.CL].

114 *This is why the path* Gordon J-S, Pasvenskiene A. Human rights for robots? A literature review. *AI Ethics.* 2021 Mar 27. link .springer.com/10.1007/s43681-021-00050-7

Peters A. Rights of human and nonhuman animals: complementing the Universal Declaration of Human Rights. *AJIL Unbound.* 2018;112:355–60.

115 *At any given point* Spotlight: impact unhealthy behaviors. America's Health Rankings. United Health Foundation. 2016 Apr. americashealthrankings.org/learn/reports/spotlight-impact -unhealthy-behaviors

115　*Lack of knowledge* NPR/PBS NewsHour/Marist Poll national survey results and analysis: 2019 and New Year's resolutions. Marist Poll. 2018 Dec 28. maristpoll.marist.edu/polls/npr-pbs -newshour-marist-poll-national-survey-results-analysis-2019 -new-years-resolutions

115　*By the second week* New Year's resolution statistics (2021 up-dated). Discover Happy Habits. 2022 Feb 3. discoverhappyhab-its.com/new-years-resolution-statistics

　　Diamond D. Just 8% of people achieve their new year's resolu-tions. Here's how they do it. *Forbes.* 2013 Jan 1. forbes.com/sites/ dandiamond/2013/01/01/just-8-of-people-achieve-their-new -years-resolutions-heres-how-they-did-it

116　*These include self-injury* Cipriano A, Cella S, Cotrufo P. Non-suicidal self-injury: a systematic review. *Front Psychol.* 2017 Nov 8;8:1946.

116　*It can also be psychological* Carsrud RS. Self-handicapping be-havior: a critical review of empirical research. PhD dissertation. Biola University. 1988 May.

117　*Depending on the tests* Bravata DM, Watts SA, Keefer AL, Mad-husudhan DK, Taylor KT, Clark DM, et al. Prevalence, predic-tors, and treatment of impostor syndrome: a systematic review. *J Gen Intern Med.* 2020 Apr;35(4):1252–75.

117　*Self-destructive behaviors* Luigjes J, Lorenzetti V, de Haan S, Youssef GJ, Murawski C, Sjoerds Z, et al. Defining compulsive behavior. *Neuropsychol Rev.* 2019 Mar;29(1):4–13.

117　*At the top of the list* Schlag AK. Percentages of problem drug use and their implications for policy making: a review of the litera-ture. *Drug Sci Poli Law.* 2020 Jan 1;6:2050324520904540.

　　Calado F, Griffiths MD. Problem gambling worldwide: an up-date and systematic review of empirical research (2000–2015). *J Behav Addict.* 2016 Dec;5(4):592–613.

　　Postlethwaite A, Kellett S, Mataix-Cols D. Prevalence of hoarding disorder: a systematic review and meta-analysis. *J Affect Disord.* 2019 Sep 1;256:309–16.

　　Derbyshire KL, Grant JE. Compulsive sexual behavior: a re-view of the literature. *J Behav Addict.* 2015 Jun;4(2):37–43.

Stevens MWR, Dorstyn D, Delfabbro PH, King DL. Global prevalence of gaming disorder: a systematic review and meta-analysis. *Aust N Z J Psychiatry.* 2021 Jun 1;55(6):553–68.

Pan Y-C, Chiu Y-C, Lin Y-H. Systematic review and meta-analysis of epidemiology of internet addiction. *Neurosci Biobehav Rev.* 2020 Nov;118:612–22.

117 *These forms of harmful* Waltmann M, Herzog N, Horstmann A, Deserno L. Loss of control over eating: a systematic review of task based research into impulsive and compulsive processes in binge eating. *PsyArXiv.* 2021. psyarxiv.com/ne3aq

117 *It is estimated that 75 percent* Copen CE. Condom use during sexual intercourse among women and men aged 15–44 in the United States: 2011–2015 National Survey of Family Growth. National Health Statistics Reports. Vol. 105. National Center for Health Statistics. 2017 Aug 10. cdc.gov/nchs/data/nhsr/nhsr105.pdf

117 *half of the deaths* Akbari M, Lankarani KB, Tabrizi R, Heydari ST, Vali M, Motevalian SA, et al. The effectiveness of mass media campaigns in increasing the use of seat belts: a systematic review. *Traffic Inj Prev.* 2021 Aug 6;22(7):495–500.

117 *The ultimate form* One in 100 deaths is by suicide. World Health Organization. 2021 Jun 17. who.int/news/item/17-06-2021-one-in-100-deaths-is-by-suicide

117 *Most suicides occur* Suicide in the world: global health estimates. Report. World Health Organization. 2019. apps.who.int/iris/bitstream/handle/10665/326948/WHO-MSD-MER-19.3-eng.pdf

118 *This pervasive mental focus* Baumeister RF, Bratslavsky E, Finkenauer C, Vohs KD. Bad is stronger than good. *Rev Gen Psychol.* 2001 Dec 1;5(4):323–70.

118 *Negativity bias* Norris CJ. The negativity bias, revisited: evidence from neuroscience measures and an individual differences approach. *Soc Neurosci.* 2021 Feb;16(1):68–82.

Lazarus J. Negativity bias: an evolutionary hypothesis and an empirical programme. *Learn Motiv.* 2021 Aug 1;75:101731.

119 *fueling the Self-Destructive Force* Parfit D. Personal identity. *Philos Rev.* 1971;80(1):3–27.

120 *Your future self* Hershfield HE. The self over time. *Curr Opin Psychol.* 2019 Apr;26:72–5.

121 *The degree of closeness* Hershfield HE, Maglio SJ. When does the present end and the future begin? *J Exp Psychol Gen.* 2020 Apr;149(4):701–18.

121 *tend to accumulate* Hershfield HE, Garton MT, Ballard K, Samanez-Larkin GR, Knutson B. Don't stop thinking about tomorrow: individual differences in future self-continuity account for saving. *Judgm Decis Mak.* 2009 Jun 1;4(4):280–6.

121 *choose more ethical* Hershfield HE, Cohen TR, Thompson L. Short horizons and tempting situations: lack of continuity to our future selves leads to unethical decision making and behavior. *Organ Behav Hum Decis Process.* 2012 Mar 1;117(2):298–310.

Van Gelder J-L, Luciano EC, Weulen Kranenbarg M, Hershfield HE. Friends with my future self: longitudinal vividness intervention reduces delinquency. *Criminology.* 2015 May;53(2): 158–79.

Van Gelder J-L, Hershfield HE, Nordgren LF. Vividness of the future self predicts delinquency. *Psychol Sci.* 2013 Jun;24(6): 974–80.

Rutchick AM, Slepian ML, Reyes MO, Pleskus LN, Hershfield HE. Future self-continuity is associated with improved health and increases exercise behavior. *J Exp Psychol Appl.* 2018 Mar;24(1):72–80.

Blouin-Hudon E-MC, Pychyl TA. Experiencing the temporally extended self: initial support for the role of affective states, vivid mental imagery, and future self-continuity in the prediction of academic procrastination. *Pers Individ Dif.* 2015 Nov 1;86: 50–6.

121 *Children who were exposed* Björkenstam E, Kosidou K, Björkenstam C. Childhood household dysfunction and risk of self-harm: a cohort study of 107 518 [*sic*] young adults in Stockholm County. *Int J Epidemiol.* 2016 Apr;45(2):501–11.

Cleare S, Wetherall K, Clark A, Ryan C, Kirtley OJ, Smith M, et al. Adverse childhood experiences and hospital-treated self-harm. *Int J Environ Res Public Health*. 2018 Jun 11;15(6). dx.doi.org/10.3390/ijerph15061235

121 *for around 40 percent* Massetti GM, Hughes K, Bellis MA, Mercy J. Global perspective on ACEs. In: Asmundson GJG, editor. *Adverse Childhood Experiences: Using Evidence to Advance Research, Practice, Policy, and Prevention*. Elsevier Academic Press; 2020. pp. 209–31.

121 *as well as for half* Hughes K, Lowey H, Quigg Z, Bellis MA. Relationships between adverse childhood experiences and adult mental well-being: results from an English national household survey. *BMC Public Health*. 2016 Mar 3;16:222.

121 *60 percent of those* Forkey H, Gillespie R, Pettersen T, Spector L, Stirling J. Adverse childhood experiences and the lifelong consequences of trauma. American Academy of Pediatrics. 2014. cdn.ymaws.com/www.ncpeds.org/resource/collection/69DEAA33-A258-493B-A63F-E0BFAB6BD2CB/ttb_aces_consequences.pdf

121 *Research has shown* Petruccelli K, Davis J, Berman T. Adverse childhood experiences and associated health outcomes: a systematic review and meta-analysis. *Child Abuse Negl*. 2019 Nov; 97:104127.

121 *Furthermore, the lifelong* Heim CM, Entringer S, Buss C. Translating basic research knowledge on the biological embedding of early-life stress into novel approaches for the developmental programming of lifelong health. *Psychoneuroendocrinology*. 2019 Jul;105:123–37.

121 *In addition, such a risk* Buss C, Entringer S, Moog NK, Toepfer P, Fair DA, Simhan HN, et al. Intergenerational transmission of maternal childhood maltreatment exposure: implications for fetal brain development. *J Am Acad Child Adolesc Psychiatry*. 2017 May;56(5):373–82.

122 *Something as frequent* Astrup A, Pedersen CB, Mok PLH, Carr MJ, Webb RT. Self-harm risk between adolescence and midlife in people who experienced separation from one or both

parents during childhood. *J Affect Disord.* 2017 Jan 15;208: 582–9.

122 ***The impact of separation*** Canetti L, Bachar E, Bonne O, Agid O, Lerer B, Kaplan De-Nour A, et al. The impact of parental death versus separation from parents on the mental health of Israeli adolescents. *Compr Psychiatry.* 2000 Sep;41(5):360–8.

122 ***Another theoretical source*** Tran The J, Ansermet J-P, Magistretti P, Ansermet F. From the principle of inertia to the death drive: the influence of the second law of thermodynamics on the Freudian theory of the psychical apparatus. *Front Psychol.* 2020 Feb 28;11:325.

122 ***In theory, the Self-Destructive Force*** Servitje L. Contagion and anarchy: Matthew Arnold and the disease of modern life. In: Nixon K, Servitje L, editors. *Endemic: Essays in Contagion Theory.* Palgrave Macmillan; 2016. pp. 21–41.

123 ***Out of the ant's head*** Sheldrake M. *Entangled Life: How Fungi Make Our Worlds, Change Our Minds and Shape Our Futures.* Random House; 2020.

123 ***Who knows, it could be*** Lovelock J. *The Revenge of Gaia: Why the Earth Is Fighting Back and How We Can Still Save Humanity.* Penguin Books; 2007.

123 ***It could also be*** Peacock K. Review of *The Medea Hypothesis:* is life on earth ultimately self-destructive? *Altern J.* 2011; 37(1): 35–6.

124 ***It could be that resisting*** Bradshaw CJA, Brook BW. The Cronus hypothesis: extinction as a necessary and dynamic balance to evolutionary diversification. *J Cosmol.* 2009;2:221–9.

124 ***For starters, what we perceive*** Hoffman DD. *The Case Against Reality: How Evolution Hid the Truth from Our Eyes.* Penguin Books; 2019.

CHAPTER 10: WHEN IS ENOUGH ENOUGH?

127 ***Affluenza is a socially transmitted*** De Graaf J, Wann D, Naylor T. *Affluenza: How Overconsumption Is Killing Us—and How to Fight Back.* 1st ed. Berrett-Koehler Publishers; 2001.

127 ***Its manifestations are clear*** Shares of gross domestic product: personal consumption expenditures. FRED Economic Data. St. Louis Fed. 2021. fred.stlouisfed.org/series/DPCERE1Q156NBEA

127 ***Americans represent 4 percent*** United States self-storage market—growth, trends and forecast (2020–2025). Report. ReportLinker. 2020 Dec. reportlinker.com/p06000981/United -States-Self-Storage-Market-Growth-Trends-and-Forecast.html ?utm_source=GNW

127 ***This detrimental condition*** University of California TV series looks at clutter epidemic in middle-class american homes. UCTV. uctv.tv/RelatedContent.aspx?RelatedID=301

128 ***Those at the bottom*** De Graaf J. Affluenza: the all-consuming epidemic. *Environ Manage Health.* 2002 Jan 1;13(2):224.

128 ***Humans would need*** Hickel J. The great challenge of the 21st century is learning to consume less. This is how we can do it. World Economic Forum. 2018 May 15. weforum.org/agenda /2018/05/our-future-depends-on-consuming-less-for-a-better -world

128 ***We are, in fact, insatiable*** Unger RM. *The Religion of the Future.* Harvard University Press; 2014.

128 ***Those who indulged*** Saad G. Evolutionary consumption. *J Consum Psychol.* 2013 Jul;23(3):351–71.
   Bouissac P. Hoarding behavior: a better evolutionary account of money psychology? *Behav Brain Sci.* 2006 Apr;29(2):181–2.

129 ***Even staying in bed*** Shelton JD. The harm of "First, Do No Harm." *JAMA.* 2000;284(21):2687–8.

129 ***This happens when*** Moynihan R, Smith R. Too much medicine? Almost certainly. *BMJ.* 2002;324:859–60.
   Moynihan R, Glasziou P, Woloshin S, Schwartz L, Santa J, Godlee F. Winding back the harms of too much medicine. *BMJ.* 2013 Feb 26;346:f1271.

130   *This is seen* Doctors' consultations. OECD Data. Organisation for Economic Co-operation and Development. data.oecd.org/healthcare/doctors-consultations.htm

130   *General population data* Scarella TM, Boland RJ, Barsky AJ. Illness anxiety disorder: psychopathology, epidemiology, clinical characteristics, and treatment. *Psychosom Med.* 2019 Jun;81(5): 398–407.

131   *It has also been shown* Fink P, Ørnbøl E, Christensen KS. The outcome of health anxiety in primary care: a two-year follow-up study on health care costs and self-rated health. *PLoS One.* 2010 Mar 24;5(3):e9873.

131   *Likely because of* Berge LI, Skogen JC, Sulo G, Igland J, Wilhelmsen I, Vollset SE, et al. Health anxiety and risk of ischaemic heart disease: a prospective cohort study linking the Hordaland Health Study (HUSK) with the Cardiovascular Diseases in Norway (CVDNOR) project. *BMJ Open.* 2016 Nov 3;6(11): e012914.

131   *a 47 percent increase* Roest AM, Martens EJ, Denollet J, de Jonge P. Prognostic association of anxiety post myocardial infarction with mortality and new cardiac events: a meta-analysis. *Psychosom Med.* 2010 Jul;72(6):563–9.

131   *As a treatment for* Tyrer P. Recent advances in the understanding and treatment of health anxiety. *Curr Psychiatry Rep.* 2018 Jun 22;20(7):49.

131   *Cognitive behavioral therapy* Axelsson E, Hedman-Lagerlöf E. Cognitive behavior therapy for health anxiety: systematic review and meta-analysis of clinical efficacy and health economic outcomes. *Expert Rev Pharmacoecon Outcomes Res.* 2019 Dec;19(6): 663–76.

132   *Overtesting is often* Lam JH, Pickles K, Stanaway F, Bell KJL. Why clinicians overtest: development of a thematic framework. *BMC Health Serv Res.* 2020 Dec;20(1):1–11.

132   *It has been estimated* O'Sullivan JW, Albasri A, Nicholson BD, Perera R, Aronson JK, Roberts N, et al. Overtesting and undertesting in primary care: a systematic review and meta-analysis. *BMJ Open.* 2018 Feb 11;8(2):e018557.

132 *Family physicians have been* Van Walraven C, Cernat G, Austin PC. Effect of provider continuity on test repetition. *Clin Chem.* 2006 Dec;52(12):2219–28.

132 *In emergency rooms* Carpenter CR, Raja AS, Brown MD. Overtesting and the downstream consequences of overtreatment: implications of "preventing overdiagnosis" for emergency medicine. *Acad Emerg Med.* 2015 Dec;22(12):1484–92.

132 *Elsewhere in hospitals* Cadamuro J, Gaksch M, Wiedemann H, Lippi G, von Meyer A, Pertersmann A, et al. Are laboratory tests always needed? Frequency and causes of laboratory overuse in a hospital setting. *Clin Biochem.* 2018 Apr;54:85–91.

132 *Overtesting also occurs* Greenberg J, Green JB. Over-testing: why more is not better. *Am J Med.* 2014 May;127(5):362–3.

132 *A careful analysis* Krogsbøll LT, Jørgensen KJ, Grønhøj Larsen C, Gøtzsche PC. General health checks in adults for reducing morbidity and mortality from disease: Cochrane systematic review and meta-analysis. *BMJ.* 2012 Nov 20;345:e7191.
    Liss DT, Uchida T, Wilkes CL, Radakrishnan A, Linder JA. General health checks in adult primary care: a review. *JAMA.* 2021 Jun 8;325(22):2294–306.

133 *On many occasions* Gilbert Welch H, Schwartz L, Woloshin S. *Overdiagnosed: Making People Sick in the Pursuit of Health.* Beacon Press; 2011.

133 *This often happens with mammograms* Kowalski AE. Mammograms and mortality: how has the evidence evolved? *J Econ Perspect.* 2021 May;35(2):119–40.

133 *when imaging technologies* Pennachio DL. Full-body scans—or scams? *Med Econ.* 2002 Aug 9;79(15):62, 68, 71.

133 *In the US, a lowering* Heart disease and stroke statistics—2020 update: a report from the American Heart Association. *Circulation.* 2020;141(9): e139–596.

133 *Even more broadly* Moynihan R. Preventing overdiagnosis: the myth, the music, and the medical meeting. *BMJ.* 2015 Mar 18;350:h1370.

134 **Some salient cases** Conrad P. Medicalization: changing contours, characteristics, and contexts. In: Cockerham WC, editor. *Medical Sociology on the Move: New Directions in Theory*. Springer Netherlands; 2013. pp. 195–214.

134 **The extent of the problem** Visser SN, Danielson ML, Bitsko RH, Holbrook JR, Kogan MD, Ghandour RM, et al. Trends in the parent-report of health care provider-diagnosed and medicated attention-deficit/hyperactivity disorder: United States, 2003–2011. *J Am Acad Child Adolesc Psychiatry*. 2014 Jan 1;53(1): 34–46.

134 **At the same time** Aaron SD, Vandemheen KL, Boulet L-P, McIvor RA, Fitzgerald JM, Hernandez P, et al. Overdiagnosis of asthma in obese and nonobese adults. *CMAJ*. 2008 Nov 18;179(11):1121–31.

134 **In Australia, 18 percent** Glasziou PP, Jones MA, Pathirana T, Barratt AL, Bell KJ. Estimating the magnitude of cancer overdiagnosis in Australia. *Med J Aust*. 2020 Mar;212(4):163–8.

134 **American physicians estimate** Lyu H, Xu T, Brotman D, Mayer-Blackwell B, Cooper M, Daniel M, et al. Overtreatment in the United States. *PLoS One*. 2017 Sep 6;12(9):e0181970.

134 **As absurd as it may sound** Stahel PF, VanderHeiden TF, Kim FJ. Why do surgeons continue to perform unnecessary surgery? *Patient Saf Surg*. 2017 Jan 13;11:1.

135 **There are up to around** Leading causes of death. National Center for Health Statistics. cdc.gov/nchs/fastats/leading-causes-of-death.htm

135 **Even though this number** Deaths and mortality. National Center for Health Statistics. cdc.gov/nchs/fastats/deaths.htm

135 **Surgeons can play** Stahel et al., Why do surgeons continue to perform unnecessary surgery?
Stahel PF. *Blood, Sweat and Tears—Becoming a Better Surgeon*. TFM Publishing; 2016.

135 **This is something** Hawley P. Unneeded operating charged to surgeons. *New York Times*. 1953 Feb 17. nytimes.com/1953/02/17/archives/unneeded-operating-charged-to-surgeons.html

135 **Those for pain relief** Jonas WB, Crawford C, Colloca L, Kaptchuk TJ, Moseley B, Miller FG, et al. To what extent are surgery and invasive procedures effective beyond a placebo response? A systematic review with meta-analysis of randomised, sham controlled trials. *BMJ Open.* 2015 Dec 11;5(12):e009655.

135 **Even spinal fusions** Raabe A, Beck J, Ulrich C. Necessary or unnecessary? A critical glance on spine surgery [in German]. *Ther Umsch.* 2014 Dec;71(12):701–5.

   Srinivas SV, Deyo RA, Berger ZD. Application of "less is more" to low back pain. *Arch Intern Med.* 2012 Jul 9;172(13):1016–20.

136 **To keep up** Haynes RB. Where's the meat in clinical journals? *ACP J Club.* 1993 Nov 1;119(3):a22.

136 **A decade later** Alper BS, Hand JA, Elliott SG, Kinkade S, Hauan MJ, Onion DK, et al. How much effort is needed to keep up with the literature relevant for primary care? *J Med Libr Assoc.* 2004 Oct;92(4):429–37.

136 **Information overload** Soroya SH, Farooq A, Mahmood K, Isoaho J, Zara S-E. From information seeking to information avoidance: understanding the health information behavior during a global health crisis. *Inf Process Manag.* 2021 Mar;58(2):102440.

136 **This can in turn** Rocha YM, de Moura GA, Desidério GA, de Oliveira CH, Lourenço FD, de Figueiredo Nicolete LD. The impact of fake news on social media and its influence on health during the COVID-19 pandemic: a systematic review. *J Public Health.* 2021 Oct 9. doi.org/10.1007/s10389-021-01658-z

137 **This in turn has led** Hogle LF. Enhancement technologies and the body. *Annu Rev Anthropol.* 2005 Oct 1;34(1):695–716.

137 **Their pursuits are** Jadad AR, Enkin MW. Computers: transcending our limits? *BMJ.* 2007 Jan 6;334(Suppl 1):S8.

   Hays SA. Transhumanism. Encyclopedia Britannica. 2018 Jun 12. britannica.com/topic/transhumanism

137 **So where is the limit** Jha S. War on death. *BMJ Opinion.* BMJ. 2015 Mar 3. blogs.bmj.com/bmj/2015/03/03/saurabh-jha-war-on-death

137 *Others are emboldened* Mayer C. *Amortality: The Pleasures and Perils of Living Agelessly.* Random House; 2011.

137 *Even if we have* Pyrkov TV, Avchaciov K, Tarkhov AE, Menshikov LI, Gudkov AV, Fedichev PO. Longitudinal analysis of blood markers reveals progressive loss of resilience and predicts human lifespan limit. *Nat Commun.* 2021 May 25;12(1):2765.

138 *At that point* Miah A. A critical history of posthumanism. In: Gordijn B, Chadwick R, editors. *Medical Enhancement and Posthumanity.* Springer Netherlands; 2009. pp. 71–94.

138 *In other instances* Organisation for Economic Co-operation and Development. *Tackling Wasteful Spending on Health.* OECD Publishing; 2017. read.oecd-ilibrary.org/social-issues-migration-health /tackling-wasteful-spending-on-health_9789264266414-en

138 *In the US, the leader* Berwick DM, Hackbarth AD. Eliminating waste in US health care. *JAMA.* 2012 Apr 11;307(14):1513–6.

138 *Driven by the need* Organisation for Economic Co-operation and Development, *Tackling Wasteful Spending on Health.*

138 *It spread quickly* Grimshaw JM, Patey AM, Kirkham KR, Hall A, Dowling SK, Rodondi N, et al. De-implementing wisely: developing the evidence base to reduce low-value care. *BMJ Qual Saf.* 2020 May;29(5):409–17.

139 *A major global concern* Dhingra S, Rahman NAA, Peile E, Rahman M, Sartelli M, Hassali MA, et al. Microbial resistance movements: an overview of global public health threats posed by antimicrobial resistance, and how best to counter. *Front Public Health.* 2020 Nov 4;8:535668.

139 *Humans are at risk* Murray CJL, Ikuta KS, Sharara F, Swetschinski L, Robles Aguilar G, Gray A, et al. Global burden of bacterial antimicrobial resistance in 2019: a systematic analysis. *Lancet.* 2022 Feb 12;399(10325):629–55.

140 *Insatiability is also seen* Wiedmann T, Lenzen M, Keyßer LT, Steinberger JK. Scientists' warning on affluence. *Nat Commun.* 2020 Jun 19. nature.com/articles/s41467-020-16941-y.pdf

140 *Such materials will likely* Choosing Wisely for Better Healthcare. Video. Consumer Reports. consumerreports.org/video/view

/healthy-living/patient-safety/2142290539001/choosing-wisely
-for-better-healthcare

Born KB, Levinson W. Choosing Wisely campaigns globally:
a shared approach to tackling the problem of overuse in healthcare. *J Gen Fam Med.* 2019 Jan;20(1):9–12.

140   *In questioning* Treharne T, Papanikitas A. Defining and detect-
ing fake news in health and medicine reporting. *J R Soc Med.*
2020 Aug 1;113(8):302–5.

140   *misinformation that is deliberately* Kanekar AS, Thombre A.
Fake medical news: avoiding pitfalls and perils. *Fam Med Community Health.* 2019 Oct 1;7(4):e000142.

142   *The main source* Soosalu G, Henwood S, Deo A. Head, heart, and
gut in decision making: development of a multiple brain preference
questionnaire. *SAGE Open.* 2019 Jan 1;9(1):2158244019837439.

Vadigepalli R, Schwaber JS. Mapping the little brain at the
heart by an interdisciplinary systems biology team. *iScience.* 2021
May 21;24(5):102433.

142   *Although these signals* Bechara A, Damasio H, Tranel D, Damasio AR. Deciding advantageously before knowing the advantageous strategy. *Science.* 1997 Feb 28;275(5304):1293–5.

Kandasamy N, Garfinkel SN, Page L, Hardy B, Critchley HD,
Gurnell M, et al. Interoceptive ability predicts survival on a London trading floor. *Sci Rep.* 2016 Sep 19;6:32986.

Sutton PA, Hornby ST, Vimalachandran D, McNally S. In-
stinct, intuition and surgical decision-making. *Bull R Coll Surg
Engl.* 2015 Sep;97(8):345–7.

CHAPTER 11: SURVIVING THE MEDICAL INDUSTRIAL COMPLEX

144   *It is often said* Osberg L, editor. *The Economic Implications of Social Cohesion.* University of Toronto Press; 2003.

Adams O, Chauhan TS, Buske L. Assessing the prospects for
physician supply and demand in Canada: wishing it was rocket
science. *Healthc Manage Forum.* 2017 Jul;30(4):181–6.

144 *In the US alone* Ambulatory care use and physician office visits. National Center for Health Statistics. cdc.gov/nchs/fastats/physician-visits.htm

144 *A survey of* Francis G. A life of pain: the average Brit suffers 5,000 injuries in a lifetime. *Iceni Magazine.* icenimagazine.co.uk/life-pain-average-brit-suffers-5000-injuries-lifetime

145 *The limited literature* Jeffery R. Normal rubbish: deviant patients in casualty departments. *Sociol Health Illn.* 1979 Jun;1(1):90–107.

Stimson GV. General practitioners, "trouble" and types of patients. *Sociol Rev.* 1974 May;22(Suppl 1):43–60.

Sointu E. "Good" patient/"bad" patient: clinical learning and the entrenching of inequality. *Sociol Health Illn.* 2017 Jan;39(1):63–77.

145 *In addition, a "traditional good patient"* Parsons T. The sick role and the role of the physician reconsidered. *Milbank Mem Fund Q Health Soc.* 1975 Summer;53(3):257–78.

Burnham JC. Why sociologists abandoned the sick role concept. *Hist Human Sci.* 2014 Feb 1;27(1):70–87.

Proulx K, Jacelon C. Dying with dignity: the good patient versus the good death. *Am J Hosp Palliat Care.* 2004 Mar;21(2):116–20.

145 *This reflects the fact* Armstrong D. Actors, patients and agency: a recent history. *Sociol Health Illn.* 2014 Feb;36(2):163–74.

145 *More modern perspectives* Miles JK. Taking patient virtue seriously. *Theor Med Bioeth.* 2019 Apr;40(2):141–9.

145 *Clinicians also regard* Parsons, The sick role.

145 *Those who do not conform* Mason D. Is "firing" the patient an unintended consequence of value-based payment? *JAMA Forum.* 2016 Feb 10;A5(1). jamanetwork.com/channels/health-forum/fullarticle/2760183

146 *This turned out to be* Jadad AR, Rizo CA, Enkin MW. I am a good patient, believe it or not. *BMJ.* 2003;326(7402):1293–95.

146 *They have since* Ellis A. The BMJ patient issue. *BMJ.* 2003 Jul 1;327(Suppl S1). bmj.com/content/327/Suppl_S1/0307221

146   *It only takes* Rizo CA, Jadad AR, Enkin M. What's a good doctor and how do you make one? Doctors should be good companions for people. *BMJ.* 2002 Sep 28;325(7366):711.

146   *This is a phenomenon* Judson TJ, Detsky AS, Press MJ. Encouraging patients to ask questions: how to overcome "white-coat silence." *JAMA.* 2013 Jun 12;309(22):2325–6.

146   *especially when dealing with* Berry LL, Danaher TS, Beckham D, Awdish RLA, Mate KS. When patients and their families feel like hostages to health care. *Mayo Clin Proc.* 2017 Sep;92(9): 1373–81.

146   *It is made worse* Irving G, Neves AL, Dambha-Miller H, Oishi A, Tagashira H, Verho A, et al. International variations in primary care physician consultation time: a systematic review of 67 countries. *BMJ Open.* 2017 Nov 8;7(10):e017902.

147   *In half of all encounters* Singh Ospina N, Phillips KA, Rodriguez-Gutierrez R, Castaneda-Guarderas A, Gionfriddo MR, Branda ME, et al. Eliciting the patient's agenda—secondary analysis of recorded clinical encounters. *J Gen Intern Med.* 2019 Jan;34(1):36–40.

147   *Surprisingly, when you* Cape J. Consultation length, patient-estimated consultation length, and satisfaction with the consultation. *Br J Gen Pract.* 2002 Dec;52(485):1004–6.

147   *Making a list* Jadad AR. Asking patients to write lists: randomised controlled trials support it. *BMJ.* 1995 Sep 16;311(7007): 746.

147   *The effects seem to be* Bottacini A, Goss C, Mazzi MA, Ghilardi A, Buizza C, Molino A, et al. The involvement of early stage breast cancer patients during oncology consultations in Italy: a multi-centred, randomized controlled trial of a question prompt sheet versus question listing. *BMJ Open.* 2017 Aug 11;7(8): e015079.

147   *Your role may change* Butow PN, Maclean M, Dunn SM, Tattersall MH, Boyer MJ. The dynamics of change: cancer patients' preferences for information, involvement and support. *Ann Oncol.* 1997 Sep;8(9):857–63.

147   *Alternatively, you might choose* O'Grady L, Jadad A. Shifting
      from shared to collaborative decision making: a change in think-
      ing and doing. *J Particip Med*. 2010;2(13):1–6.

      Caridi family, Poduri A, Devinsky O, Tabacinic M, Jadad AR.
      Experiencing positive health, as a family, while living with a rare
      complex disease: bringing participatory medicine through collab-
      orative decision making into the real world. *J Particip Med*.
      2020;12(2):e17602.

148   *There is a significant* Flynn KE, Smith MA, Vanness D. A typol-
      ogy of preferences for participation in healthcare decision mak-
      ing. *Soc Sci Med*. 2006 Sep;63(5):1158–69.

      Singh JA, Sloan JA, Atherton PJ, Smith T, Hack TF,
      Huschka MM, et al. Preferred roles in treatment decision making
      among patients with cancer: a pooled analysis of studies using the
      Control Preferences Scale. *Am J Manag Care*. 2010 Sep;16(9):
      688–96.

148   *Nevertheless, although it* Noteboom EA, May AM, van der
      Wall E, de Wit NJ, Helsper CW. Patients' preferred and perceived
      level of involvement in decision making for cancer treatment: a
      systematic review. *Psychooncology*. 2021 Oct;30(10):1663–79.

148   *Commonly, you will* Tariman JD, Berry DL, Cochrane B,
      Doorenbos A, Schepp K. Preferred and actual participation roles
      during health care decision making in persons with cancer: a sys-
      tematic review. *Ann Oncol*. 2010 Jun;21(6):1145–51.

148   *Whenever you enter* Twomey M, Sammon D, Nagle T. Memory
      recall/information retrieval challenges within the medical ap-
      pointment: a review of the literature. *J Decis Syst*. 2020 Jul
      2;29(3):148–81.

148   *The more information* Kessels RPC. Patients' memory for medi-
      cal information. *J R Soc Med*. 2003 May;96(5):219–22.

148   *In fact, 40 to 80 percent* McGuire LC. Remembering what the
      doctor said: organization and adults' memory for medical infor-
      mation. *Exp Aging Res*. 1996 Oct;22(4):403–28.

      Anderson JL, Dodman S, Kopelman M, Fleming A. Patient
      information recall in a rheumatology clinic. *Rheumatol Rehabil*.
      1979 Feb;18(1):18–22.

148   *Scientific evidence also* Berkman ND, Sheridan SL, Dona-
      hue KE, Halpern DJ, Crotty K. Low health literacy and health
      outcomes: an updated systematic review. *Ann Intern Med.* 2011
      Jul 19;155(2):97–107.
          Mantwill S, Monestel-Umaña S, Schulz PJ. The relationship
      between health literacy and health disparities: a systematic re-
      view. *PLoS One.* 2015 Dec 23;10(12):e0145455.

149   *It has been shown that each* Sentell T, Zhang W, Davis J,
      Baker KK, Braun KL. The influence of community and individ-
      ual health literacy on self-reported health status. *J Gen Intern
      Med.* 2014 Feb;29(2):298–304.

149   *Stress and anxiety* Nguyen MH, Smets EMA, Bol N, Bron-
      ner MB, Tytgat KMAJ, Loos EF, et al. Fear and forget: how anxi-
      ety impacts information recall in newly diagnosed cancer patients
      visiting a fast-track clinic. *Acta Oncol.* 2019 Feb;58(2):182–8.

149   *This is likely* Jansen J, van Weert J, van der Meulen N, van Dul-
      men S, Heeren T, Bensing J. Recall in older cancer patients: mea-
      suring memory for medical information. *Gerontologist.* 2008
      Apr;48(2):149–57.

149   *Getting information verbally* Hoek AE, Anker SCP, van Beeck EF,
      Burdorf A, Rood PPM, Haagsma JA. Patient discharge instruc-
      tions in the emergency department and their effects on compre-
      hension and recall of discharge instructions: a systematic review
      and meta-analysis. *Ann Emerg Med.* 2020 Mar 1;75(3):435–44.

149   *It has been shown, consistently* Watson PWB, McKinstry B. A
      systematic review of interventions to improve recall of medical
      advice in healthcare consultations. *J R Soc Med.* 2009 Jun;102(6):
      235–43.

149   *Involving trusted people* Laidsaar-Powell RC, Butow PN, Bu S,
      Charles C, Gafni A, Lam WWT, et al. Physician-patient-
      companion communication and decision-making: a systematic
      review of triadic medical consultations. *Patient Educ Couns.* 2013
      Apr 1;91(1):3–13.

150   *For that reason* Bickerstaffe S. Towards whole person care. Re-
      port. Institute for Public Policy Research. 2013 Dec. ippr.org/

files/images/media/files/publication/2013/11/whole-person
-care_Dec2013_11518.pdf

150 *When this is done well* Continuity and coordination of care: a
practice brief to support implementation of the WHO Framework on integrated people-centred health services. World Health
Organization. 2018. apps.who.int/iris/bitstream/handle/10665
/274628/9789241514033-eng.pdf?ua=1

150 *A very practical* Buja A, Francesconi P, Bellini I, Barletta V, Gi-
rardi G, Braga M, et al. Health and health service usage outcomes
of case management for patients with long-term conditions: a review of reviews. *Prim Health Care Res Dev.* 2020 Aug 3;21:e26.

Øvretveit J. Evidence: does clinical coordination improve
quality and save money? Report. Vol. 1. The Health Foundation.
2011.

150 *Such a person* Wise J. Patients must have single point of contact
for care needs, says think tank. *BMJ.* 2013 Dec 3;347:f7202.

151 *Second opinions are usually* Hillen MA, Medendorp NM,
Daams JG, Smets EMA. Patient-driven second opinions in oncology: a systematic review. *Oncologist.* 2017 Oct;22(10):
1197–211.

Burger PM, Westerink J, Vrijsen BEL. Outcomes of second
opinions in general internal medicine. *PLoS One.* 2020 Jul
9;15(7):e0236048.

Olver I, Carey M, Bryant J, Boyes A, Evans T, Sanson-Fisher R.
Second opinions in medical oncology. *BMC Palliat Care.* 2020
Jul 21;19(1):112.

151 *Requesting a second opinion* Ruetters D, Keinki C, Schroth S,
Liebl P, Huebner J. Is there evidence for a better health care for
cancer patients after a second opinion? A systematic review.
J Cancer Res Clin Oncol. 2016 Jul;142(7):1521–8.

Könsgen N, Prediger B, Bora A-M, Glatt A, Hess S, Weißflog
V, et al. Analysis of second opinion programs provided by German statutory and private health insurance—a survey of statutory
and private health insurers. *BMC Health Serv Res.* 2021 Mar
9;21(1):209.

151 **with almost 60 percent** Heeg E, Civil YA, Hillen MA, Smorenburg CH, Woerdeman LAE, Groen EJ, et al. Impact of second opinions in breast cancer diagnostics and treatment: a retrospective analysis. *Ann Surg Oncol.* 2019 Dec;26(13):4355–63.

151 **In addition, up to** Greenfield G, Shmueli L, Harvey A, Quezada-Yamamoto H, Davidovitch N, Pliskin JS, et al. Patient-initiated second medical consultations—patient characteristics and motivating factors, impact on care and satisfaction: a systematic review. *BMJ Open.* 2021 Sep 1;11(9):e044033.

151 **Only one-third** Weyerstraß J, Prediger B, Neugebauer E, Pieper D. Second opinions before surgery have the potential to reduce costs—an exploratory analysis. *Z Orthop Unfall.* 2021 Aug; 159(4):406–11.

152 **A careful assessment** Graboys TB, Biegelsen B, Lampert S, Blatt CM, Lown B. Results of a second-opinion trial among patients recommended for coronary angiography. *JAMA.* 1992 Nov 11;268(18):2537–40.

152 **The main issue** Nabhan M, Elraiyah T, Brown DR, Dilling J, LeBlanc A, Montori VM, et al. What is preventable harm in healthcare? A systematic review of definitions. *BMC Health Serv Res.* 2012 May 25;12(1):128.

152 **An extensive analysis of** Panagioti M, Khan K, Keers RN, Abuzour A, Phipps D, Kontopantelis E, et al. Prevalence, severity, and nature of preventable patient harm across medical care settings: systematic review and meta-analysis. *BMJ.* 2019 Jul 17;366. bmj.com/content/366/bmj.l4185

153 **It can be linked** Jadad AR. Facing leadership that kills. *J Public Health Policy.* 2021;42:651–7.

153 **Nevertheless, they can** Wright J, Lawton R, O'Hara J, Armitage G, Sheard L, Marsh C, et al. Improving patient safety through the involvement of patients: development and evaluation of novel interventions to engage patients in preventing patient safety incidents and protecting them against unintended harm. NIHR Journals Library; 2016. europepmc.org/article/nbk/nbk390627

153 *It might also be beneficial* Chegini Z, Arab-Zozani M, Shariful Islam SM, Tobiano G, Abbasgholizadeh Rahimi S. Barriers and facilitators to patient engagement in patient safety from patients and healthcare professionals' perspectives: a systematic review and meta-synthesis. *InNursing Forum*. 2021;56(4):938–49.

153 *Despite being a proven* Melville NA. WHO hand-hygiene initiative largely ignored. *Medscape*. 2011 May 20. medscape.com/viewarticle/743111

153 *Twenty-one percent of hand* Cobb TK. Wrong site surgery—where are we and what is the next step? *Hand*. 2012 Jun;7(2):229–32.

154 *Matching what you need* Jadad AR, Arango A, Sepúlveda JD, Espinal S, Rodríguez D, Wind K, editors. *Unleashing a Pandemic of Health from the Workplace: Believing Is Seeing*. Beati; 2017.

155 *These diseases affect* Chen S, Kuhn M, Prettner K, Bloom DE. The macroeconomic burden of noncommunicable diseases in the United States: estimates and projections. *PLoS One*. 2018 Nov 1;13(11):e0206702.

155 *The most common* Raghupathi W, Raghupathi V. An empirical study of chronic diseases in the United States: a visual analytics approach to public health. *Int J Environ Res Public Health*. 2018 Mar 1;15(3):431.

156 *This rate keeps increasing* Habib SH, Saha S. Burden of noncommunicable disease: global overview. *Diabetes Metab Syndr: Clin Res*. 2010 Jan 1;4(1):41–7.

156 *Chronic diseases are also* Galenkamp H, Braam AW, Huisman M, Deeg DJH. Seventeen-year time trend in poor self-rated health in older adults: changing contributions of chronic diseases and disability. *Eur J Public Health*. 2013 Jun;23(3):511–7.

156 *Most people (80 percent)* Iezzoni LI. Multiple chronic conditions and disabilities: implications for health services research and data demands. *Health Serv Res*. 2010 Oct;45(5 Pt 2):1523–40.

156 *Half of the patients* Terner M, Reason B, McKeag AM, Tipper B, Webster G. Chronic conditions more than age drive health system use in Canadian seniors. *Healthc Q*. 2011;14(3):19–22.

156 *Thus, many people* Wastesson JW, Morin L, Tan ECK, Johnell K. An update on the clinical consequences of polypharmacy in older adults: a narrative review. *Expert Opin Drug Saf.* 2018 Dec; 17(12):1185–96.

Morin L, Johnell K, Laroche M-L, Fastbom J, Wastesson JW. The epidemiology of polypharmacy in older adults: register-based prospective cohort study. *Clin Epidemiol.* 2018 Mar 12;10: 289–98.

156 *All of these "solutions"* Scibona P, Beruto MV, Savoy NE, Simonovich VA. Polypharmacy and the older patient: the clinical pharmacologist perspective. In: Musso CG, Jauregui JR, Macías-Núñez JF, Covic A, editors. *Frailty and Kidney Disease: A Practical Guide to Clinical Management.* Springer International; 2021. pp. 91–104.

156 *Piling on* Halli-Tierney AD, Scarbrough C, Carroll D. Polypharmacy: evaluating risks and deprescribing. *Am Fam Physician.* 2019 Jul 1;100(1):32–8.

157 *A review of multiple studies* Page AT, Clifford RM, Potter K, Schwartz D, Etherton-Beer CD. The feasibility and effect of deprescribing in older adults on mortality and health: a systematic review and meta-analysis. *Br J Clin Pharmacol.* 2016 Sep; 82(3):583–623.

158 *We tried to gain insights* Zaman M, Andoniou E, Wind K, Gibson J, Upshur R, Rojas G, et al. A good death: non-negotiable personal conditions for clinicians, healthcare administrators and support staff. *BMJ Support Palliat Care.* 2021 Apr 12. spcare.bmj .com/content/early/2021/04/11/bmjspcare-2020-002878.long (abstract only)

Zaman M, Espinal-Arango S, Mohapatra A, Jadad AR. What would it take to die well? A systematic review of systematic reviews on the conditions for a good death. *The Lancet Healthy Longevity.* 2021 Sep 1;2(9):e593–600.

CHAPTER 12: YOU ARE A FORMIDABLE MARVEL

168 *One option was discovered* Epictetus, The Enchiridion. Carter E, translator classics.mit.edu/Epictetus/epicench.html

168   *It is known as* Striker G. Ataraxia: happiness as tranquillity. *Monist.* 1990;73(1):97–110.

168   *Along the same lines* Han-Pile B. Nietzsche and amor fati. *Eur J Philos.* 2011 Jun;19(2):224–61.

169   *You can dissolve* Ackoff R. *Differences.* Triarchy Press; 2010.

ALEX JADAD, MD DPhil FRCPC FCAHS FRSA LLD, is a physician, philosopher, educator, researcher, entrepreneur, author and innovator. He is a pioneer of evidence-based medicine and digital health, and the creator of the Jadad scale, the most widely used tool to assess clinical trial quality worldwide. Alex leads large-scale efforts to shape the future of health and medicine, and is an adviser to heads of states and multinational corporations. He also holds a doctor of philosophy degree from Balliol College at the University of Oxford.

TAMEN JADAD-GARCIA is an entrepreneur and philosopher who builds businesses and leads strategic projects with Fortune 500 companies in healthcare, consumer goods, and technology. Tamen is also the author of scientific articles and books spanning end-of-life care, love, and the future of health. She received her honors degree in business management from King's College London.

ABOUT THE TYPE

This book was set in Garamond, a typeface originally designed by the Parisian type cutter Claude Garamond (c. 1500–61). This version of Garamond was modeled on a 1592 specimen sheet from the Egenolff-Berner foundry, which was produced from types assumed to have been brought to Frankfurt by the punch cutter Jacques Sabon (c. 1520–80).

Claude Garamond's distinguished romans and italics first appeared in *Opera Ciceronis* in 1543–44. The Garamond types are clear, open, and elegant.